Hyper mania revealed

Surviving Hyper Mania in your life and the life of those around you

By Sushi I Toy

Published by
Chipmunkapublishing
PO Box 6872
Brentwood
Essex CM13 1ZT
United Kingdom

First published 2005
Second edition 2007

Copyright © 2007 Chipmunkapublishing

A record of this book is in the British Library.

ISBN 190469781X

http://www.chipmunkapublishing.com

Forward

Have you ever wondered what drives Richard Branson? Why Ryanair is growing? Or Easyjet has so many sister companies?

This book gives insight into the types of people that make them work. Some are in-your-face and some are behind the scenes. By the end of the book you will be able to spot these people. Think like them when you have to and be the real you.
Anyone who slows them down "does not get it."

Mania gives you edge over the competition, mortals just crumble.

There are four sections within the book: hyper mania described covers the medical aspects of the condition; hyper mania in personal life, once you understand the person we can then talk about the condition, covers the 24/7 of a hyper maniac, you will see that his home life is often different and understand why. This covers a real hyper maniac that lives the trails, highs and lows. For the last two, hyper mania in business covers the working and pure money making machine of a hyper maniac. You could increase your income or life style by following these rules. I am a hyper maniac what now? covers the next step.

You have to start somewhere, expect the unexpected.

Dedication

To all those that understand I give you power, to those who do not, you still don't get it.

To my parents, my environment and contacts, you made me what I am today.

Book one: hyper mania described

What is the purpose of this book?
Everything has a purpose, this book's purpose is to challenge **YOU,** the reader.
People with hyper mania or Hypomania are more likely to do what they have to do, rather than what they want to do.

Until it finally sinks in, you will usually find your failure is based on your hard headed experience. You succeed in business because you failed five times before.

You have to learn, and here you will.

This book is intended to reveal the inner thoughts of hyper mania and hypomania, [you will either be interested or not.) [omit? Obvious point]

For those who want to develop themselves or **understand for** others it will be an interesting read. For those that can't understand go and buy Harry Potter. Because people that don't get it slow hyper maniacs and hypomaniacs down.

You can do so much more and if you want to, this is the book for you. If not, carry on with your life and expect no more that you get. Do you want to start understanding yourself?

You will reap what you sow, <u>challenge everything</u>.
Expect nothing.

The world is changing, you need to evolve or die out. This book is intended to help you start to evolve. But for you to evolve, you must start to understand.

People with hyper mania or hypo mania are more likely to do what they have to do, rather than what they want to do.

Until it finally sinks in. You will usually find your failure is based on your hard headed [what? Doesn't make sense].

You might get an Underlying trend of NLP (Neuro-linguistic Programming), it's what a good maniac uses.

Ever questioned why you do what you want to rather than what you have to?

Ever wanted to do more?

It is here and more…………..

Hyper mania and Hypo mania

The dictionary describes hyper mania as excessive enthusiasm (inward) while hypo maniac is expressed in a more outward way (in-your-face).

A medical professional would describe it as a state of mind characterised by excessive cheerfulness and increased activity.

I would just say it's a rollercoaster.

My thanks to John D Gartner and his book, The Hypo manic edge, ISBN 0743243447. Helping give me the two extremes, both of which I have suffered.

This book helped me define the divide between hypo maniac and a hyper maniac.

They are similar by:

The biggest single effect is that they are **not afraid of death.**

Conversion; the dreams are a theme to the maniac. While often dreams are forgotten within ten minutes of waking the maniac can remember more dreams. The hyper will have dreams of power while the hypo will have dreams of doing. Some of these dreams might not come true for ten years. Just like déjà-vus.

Hypomania and hypermania are mild forms of mania, the hypomaniac being full of drive, confidence and great plans, while the hypermaniacs think in logical patterns. They know where they have to go and get there in baby steps.

This is not a condition you could be locked up for. There is no medication for it, while being similar is not the same as being Bi-Polar.

Hypo: the charismatic leader
Hyper: behind that leader

Hypos talk fast, think fast and act fast.
Hyper, talk slow (do you get it?), think fast and act according to demands.

Bi polars and maniacs can reach denial, this is key as this often acts as an away [a way?]for them to overcome the obstacle.

Both hide pain although this is more visible in hypomaniacs as they are in the lime light.

Both know good ideas when they see one, hypers and hypos are not exclusive, you can progress between them, often a progression from hypo to hyper is normal.

Hypo

Hypos are self centred, me, me, me. Hypo maniacs think big, create the dots and then someone else has to join them.

Often found playing around with the opposite sex, very high sex drive. They live life in the fast lane.

Hyper

Hypers are sure of their direction and get there by baby steps. They consider their close contacts and might even make a detour, to help someone they trust.

The hypers will undermine by quoting facts, which are the key defence and act like mud (slowing down) because the opposition will not expect it. They will then talk to each advisor to win them over, rather than a frontal assault on a group.

The standard response is to move faster, get aggressive, pile on the energy: a frontal assault on the opposing force.

Hypers created A) and B), then race there. However it's a one-horse race: them.

They are found in very safe relationships, stable environments with stable family life. They tend to look after others more.

However, they are still a **coiled spring**.

While not being a doctor myself, seeing a medical view of hypo maniac and being a hyper maniac myself, this book confirms what I had known for over twenty years. There are still few people who understand either. Both inside and outside of the medical profession.

These people are focused to learn and overact, if they do not know the subject this time, they will next time. Just watch out. Do they use disinformation, divide and conquer or something equally nasty?

They do have a built NLP . Within most people it's an optional extra. Or some do not use it at all.

Eye contact is treated differently; one will stare until you submit, the other will use it where they need to.

They come in two flavours, in-your-face and stealth. Watch out for the stealth ones as they are really special and in control.

Ask yourself these questions:

1. If someone is in your way, will you knock them over?
2. Are you the life and soul of the party?
3. Do you need less than 6 hours sleep?

In-your-face (Hypo maniac)

They will invade your personal space and sit eyeball to eyeball in front of you until you submit. They are very good at negotiation and discussion; their fast reflexes enable them to process data quicker (they do have extra high IQ and even more cunningly - emotional intelligence).

On the phone you have to say yes, because they force you to do so. This is similar to people with other medical conditions like Aspergers> However, these are the sharpest of the bunch. Sure they have their down days but even they are hard for the average person.

They have a lower amount of planning due to the pressure that they put on people. However this is how they get things done; they see the higher level.

Most have inbuilt desire to share information (unlike the stealth), they have high trust and at times can resort to physical violence or outbursts.

They are the people you can see, they are in-your-face until you submit.

This type of hyper maniac often creates the environment as atmosphere, more often as tension, (to be discussed later.)

Stealth (Hyper maniac)

Ask yourself these questions:
- If someone is in your way, will you have a planned way round them?
- In a party are you looking at other people's interaction?
- Do you need less than 6 hours sleep?
- Do you use sleep to plan?

Lock up your daughter and your mouth. A different animal but the same family. They take in the data and feed it back in such a way that you have to follow them.

These are the quiet ones, always thinking and planning, then pouncing like a coiled spring.

They are often found beside the hypomaniac (or two at the same time) you have to know what to look out for - as they are hard to spot. They are so cunning, but they do pay attention to details and join up the dots.

They get to know their contacts' patterns, down to eating and drinking times. They can sense the tension on a phone call. Within companies, expect them to know the inner movements within a short period of time. Even in conversations they can read body language and move the conversation without needing to know the local tongue.

They are very trustworthy, they have high respect and HATE fools. They tend to keep their own council and blend in. Boys blend in and plan because they know that planning and preparation is everything. They are results driven, but they target their results, to the outcome they want.

This is the enemy you can't see until it's too late. They are the people you can't see coming while the in-your-face you can see a mile off, this type might be right next to you. In military campaigns they are best described as sleepers.

It is best to have them on your team; they need to have faith in you.

You will not see these people, they do not stick out and they are often found behind someone.

They could be a good **FD**, [?}hiding behind a **CEO.** They gather information on so many different levels. The only clue to find one might be that most people consider these people as sad gits. They understand and can apply Six Sigma, TQM, Fiscal 2 along with other work practices, discussed later in the book. They are good at reasoning on many levels and talking to all classes at their own level. However not the life a soul of the party, but people look up to them.

They use disinformation, just like the prisoner in the 1960's cult program. They might learn a subject for later and I mean ten years later. They can spot future trends and add to their skill set at any time.

This type feeds off the environment and atmosphere, often uses Jedi powers to sense the forthcoming debate or mood swings, discussed later. They appear more laid back, because they lull you into a false sense of security. Some call this perception, but the reality is that you open up more and this gives them more data to use against you.

They both know what they want and how they are going to get there. It's the same journey, however by different directions. The lack of fear within-your-face is so strong, they are just like a bull elephant.

Do not try and use or abuse these people, you will be the victim.

Bi polar

The dictionary describes bi polar as two extremes.

A medical professional would describe it as an euphoric mood that changes rapidly to irritability where thought and speech are rapid to the point of incoherence and connections between ideas may be hard to follow. Treatment is usually done with drugs such as lithium or phenothiazines. They suffer episodes of depression and mania.

Bi polar type one: classically depressed

Bi polar type two: mood swings, highs and lows

I would just say it's a **trainee** hyper maniac and very bright.

I know a number of bipolars and they are great people, but they are very much in-your-face. They demand a great deal in time and effort. I would rather be with a group of people affected by bipolar than most other groups.

They are very bright, anyone that has read *A Can of Madness* by Jason Pegler will see what the life of a bi polar can do.

Some people I know have this condition but are unable to control it (more later in the book.)

The bi polar person has high and low days. They are often given medication to control the mood swings. However a simple monitor of food and drink intake takes the lows out.

Their thirst for knowledge is vast, they will read and do anything. I do mean anything.

They are very good salesmen, similar to the in-your-face hyper mania people.

Bi polar people have what's called mania, when they are stable ask them what to do. When they are down you can help them.

This is a proven medical condition **unlike** hyper mania and hypo mania.

Physical and Mental health

Both the physical and mental are so related it's hard to keep them apart. The more of the right food you eat the better your body is. You can't do a full presentation after a heavy night on the beer.

Mental health is going to be the second highest global killer from 2020 according to The World health organisation.

The number of external factors that influence mental health are increasing. As the McDonald's generation, PlayStation generation and pill popping generation take over, the world becomes a harder place to live in. This creates social disorder, as they can't communicate and find physical activities hard to do.

A simple example is stress. Let's say that you have children and they play up. How do you deal with that stress? Kick the cat? Red wine? Weed? Walk in the garden? Hit them?

But if this stress goes on too long the impact is going to change you.

You are what you eat

It's true: you are conditioning your body, therefore that thing they call a balanced diet is critical to keeping your body in trim. Both mind and body depend on what goes into your mouth. Therefore as discussed later, a poor diet can lead to lack of energy. The mind will start slipping and it could cost you your job or even your life.

They say two can live as cheap as one, however this is not about food but rather mental stimulation.

There is a delicate balance in all you eat or drink; too much coconut milk can produce the runs. While not enough vitamin C, produces sore gums, teeth and lips. To be at your peak you need a balanced diet.

The caffeine- based drinks within young people are very scary. In clubs there is low alcohol and increase sales of caffeine products lead to greater highs.[sentence unclear] However this is at a cost to the person. How do you take someone down who has had too much caffeine? Hospitals near the big nightclubs in Spain are finding out.

The new replacement to E is Special K, this puts people in a trance and gives a different Kick. However it tends to kill more brain cells than E or cannabis.

Too much or too little sugar can kill. There have been many cases of people being hyperglycaemic all over the world. This creates all sorts of stress in the body, which in some cases leads to the body burning out.
Your body has natural chemicals, like lithium, iron, water etc with out these you will shortly die.
Look after your body, you only get one.

Chipmunka do an amazing video of how schizophrenics handle their condition by drumming or meditation. You can control your body without external drugs, it's called NLP.

If you have seen *Super Size Me*, the food was (in large amounts) not good for him. We live in an age where we spend less time eating. Food preparation is a chore and washing up not on the agenda.

Go to the developed world where eating is part of the culture; in Italy a meal could take 3 hours. Better than the 2-4 minutes that the fast food chains allow.

However 50 years ago, families sat down at a table. Yes, table, the thing that you sit at in PROPER food restaurants. Without TV, there was interaction and conversation. Now you will eat, in front of the TV, something that's been prepared en masse and blasted in the microwave. TV dinners have been designed by the TV companies to keep you there in front of the TV.

Go on a holiday, on a desert island and you will eat freshly prepared food without additives. You will focus on life and not the TV. Your mood set will also change, with no external demands you will de-stress and feel happy.

Stress junkies are to be avoided at all costs. They feed on stress and give it to others.

The Times newspaper in the UK reported that Britain counts £100Bn as for the cost of stress in the work place (May 16th 2005). The article goes on to explain that the poor relationships, including low levels of trust, lack of supportiveness and no one that listens, along with long shifts, bad travel and work overload or under load all build up to produce stress.

The facts and figures have been supplied by a mind report. This is the tip of the iceberg; the balance is as always delicate. This is why the report refers to work overload and work under load.

Work overload is easy to explain, however under load is best explained as "I am Bored".

There will always be those people taking a sick day or bunking off but here will be hard workers too. In Japan you have no power, but if you are not at your desk for eight hours a day you are laid off.

The UK has become a 24/7 way of living, you can shop at a supermarket from 8 am Monday to 10 pm Saturday. I like shopping between midnight and 6 am, it's empty of people and they have real staff during these hours.

Anyone who has watched Sky programmes like "Paul Mckenna's I can change your life" will see that the process deals with the psychical and the mental. They are both interlinked in such a way and dealing with one can create an imbalance.

Perception & reality

Perception is described as process for each of the senses by identifying the environmental stimuli, sensory receptors and path of sensation.

Reality is more tactile (but only just.)

The Magic Circle use deception (or was that deception) and it is only when you see how the trick is done that it becomes reality.

In a more down to earth example the perception can be described as: there are two men, one with a Rolex watch, an Audi TT and a four-bedroom house, long drive and pool. One with no watch, a ten-year old car and a four-bedroom house.

Reality is painful.

Does the first have more debits than assets, the second owes no one. Or the other way round. Which one is happier with his lot?

You might meet someone and think that they have it all but really they owe it all and are unhappy to boot.

It's the hyper maniac that has everything; he knows when to change his car, while the hypo maniac has outgoings in excess or incomings.

A hyper maniac uses both, but does make sure that they are correctly used. Like a good salesman you might talk about your investments into companies but not boast. Net worth is a difficult subject. Hyper maniacs and bi polar are not normally liars, they might bend the truth but they know that they can be found out.

They are into the area of perception. You talk to an in-your-face person and they make you think that you are the centre of their universe. What is said is not as important as what was implied.

For example: on a recent trip away, the perception was not far from reality. Some wanted to believe the trip was for business and others knew it was a birthday gift. While the reality is it was both for business and pleasure.

The hyper maniac uses both of these, however they use different measure of in-your-face (more reality), because they want physical things. The stealth is about perception.

An example is in one job I had some years ago, I liked the company car and had the option of buying it. I also had another job lined up. I need to move fast. I ended up buying the car for £3500 undervalued and still leaving the employer without a clue. How? Well, I followed the law change that I had the option of a car, I found out what the company book value was and the real value. I (without being in-your-face) showed the car to be the wrong car for the company, as well as me as I paid too much tax. I then convinced the company that I needed the money rather than the car and I purchased the car. Three years later I sold the car to my brother in law for the same sum of money (also using stealth).

Hyper maniacs are 5th Dan in the arts of perception and reality. They can do what real black belts do, use the enemies' weapons against them.

How? Well, they carry on testing you.

If you say that you are a director of a company, they, hyper maniacs, do a company search, visit you or phone you up. Then if they commit to doing something, this will be followed up. Their personal database on you will be extensive, contained in grey matter.

Why do hyper maniacs push you? To undermine you and get you to submit. They will present a good story, but like the good magic man (covered later in this book) and you will be forced to look at the right hand not the left. The facts will be facts but in such a way you will be forced to admit that they did not lie. Hyper maniacs tend not to lie, they might bend the truth but they do not lie. You might be forced to lie to save yourself from commitment. Don't forget your lies come back to haunt you.

This is why they make great sales people. Use the in-your-face chap to open the door and use the Stealth to develop that relationship. The customer will go nowhere because your team would know more about the business than the clients' staff themselves.

A real example:

I was involved with a company in the North East. It was a family run company with a turnover of £35m. They sold out to London based investors and appointed a CEO. While I had only been to the company four times before change of ownership I had gathered much data. During the presentation of supply solutions to the CEO, his PA interrupted the meeting asking for an aerial shot of the building. He was new and the handover had been so quick he really did not know where any of the company files where. My reply was simple - if he could not find a copy I could supply him an image from the very laptop I was presenting from. My colleague and I had a laugh about this shortly after as whenever he required further information we received a call. His role of CEO was undermined. We knew that he was on thin ice because he did not understand the company or how it works. He did not deserve the high salary he was receiving.

Starting with you (the power of one-YOU!!)

You will have seen films like *Cry Freedom*. Anyone knowing an oppressed culture or people will understand that the vision started with one person. Martin Luther king led the black people to freedom. Could this have happened with a white middle class person? I think not.

Ghandi and Genghis Khan toured their country united to fight the oppressor or being the oppressor. [Not Clear] They started with one person, one vision.

You can reprogram yourself into a better person; I would recommend *Teach Yourself NLP*]author?]by Hodder Headline. ISBN 0340 812575

You hold the key to turn your life around. A person with a drink problem can do nothing unless he understands and admits he has a drink problem.

A nice way that a drunken woman explains her own issue is they only have a drink problem if they drink more than me and I do not like them. They are a drunkard, they see a small aspect of someone's life that is wrong, while theirs is just screwed up.

I have seen people walk on fire; I have seen minds changed forever. The power of the mind is awesome. However, historically it has sometimes been used for good, often for bad. Some are weak and some are strong, they often do it for different reasons, normally fear or greed.

But being positive often tips the balance. You will see a number of books on being positive. Even bad news can be good news told in a positive manner. Just a smile on your face when telling bad news can make a difference.

Try going home to the family with the world on your shoulders, you will find some of your own family say what is wrong, then,well I had it worst. While others steer clear of you. Go home with a smile and your conversation that evening will be much better.

The in-your-face hyper maniac has extreme highs and lows when going home, while the stealth has a level condition because they can trigger a more positive mental condition.

You have to decide to change but many are not able to, and it's even harder to keep being happy. This is all discussed further in the book, you will have a home face and work face. They tend to tell different stories, because of your environment.

We are all a little mad

Chipmunka Publishing has a strap line **"We are all a little mad",** as opposed to **you don't have to be mad to work here but it helps.**

The horror of the pure numbers is great, one in four will suffer a mental condition during their life. But you are not out of the woods yet!! These people are not in one village or town. They are mixed in, therefore these people will have contact with others bringing the number up to 3 in 4. No, I hear you say, well, yes. These people go to work, have family loved ones and contact with the outside world. These people we call councillor, careers and support workers.

Border line personality disorders group states 80% of all people have some form of personality disorder.

The numbers are too large to figure, so we are a little mad, but there is no need for drugs.

It might start with, stress at work or in the family, move on to poor eating due to lack of time, resulting in bad health then into a break down.

Baby blues too, is common in mothers that have just had a child. They can burst into tears for the smallest of reasons.

There are some good books on what can influence your mental health. It might not be you; it could be your environment.

But needless to say they can't lock us all u because we are all a little mad.

Environment, food and love

Environment is such an issue now. In some cases the government are doing a great job of keeping it as it was. In other cases enlightenment has left the building.

Follow the Chart line

Low job - low food - bad heath- low job- low money

In New Orleans people have lost everything, only just keeping alive. They will have state aid for many years or more to escape the trap.

The European governments are anti-GM crops while it's standard practice in the USA.

The old adage *'You can take a girl out of a trailer park but you can't take the trailer park out of the girl'* is true.

The natural resources of the world are running out. In the last 100 years we have used more than any other time.

We are becoming conditioned to live life faster, spend more and consume more. In the UK, landfill is such an issue, while in the developing world they feed off others' rubbish.

If your environment is upsetting you - change your environment.

If you grow up in a society that promotes sleeping around or having unprotected sex, then you move out before you become a victim of your environment. Everything is becoming consumed, not used, loved or looked after.

The middle class follow this Food chart

Own food - mass produced - organic

Your feudal farming gives way to mass production and then you look for organic in your super market.

As discussed you are what you eat, you need not be a dictated [Not clear] to work out what is good for you. You need not have those expensive pills; in fact good eating is the order of the day. You look at people who have low incomes their bodies are in better condition because they are living off the earth.

In Latvia, as an example, McDonald's lose money, not only if their product is new to the people, but it doubles a good meal in the traditional eating houses. [Not clear]

Some of the new European countries can show a thing or two to these old countries. They have practiced organic farming and not moved onto intensive farming. While everywhere else, farmers are trying to become organic because that's what the buying public ask for. The UK organic food market is increasing by 12% a year, while the margin for such a product is 20% higher than mass produced product.

There is no surprise that after the foot and mouth cases in the UK, farmers received a good payout from the state. They still wanted to be in farming however they realised that the UK was not the place to be. They sold their land at £8,000 per acre and moved to Latvia, Lithuania etc buying land for £200 per acre.
Not that they really worked on the farms but they had a low cost business under easier conditions.

Even the air you breathe is food to your body. It gives energy, however in the developing world there is an increase in asthma as the air becomes polluted. Crops contain too many nitrates and phosphates.

The size of the average European waist is on the increase and this is due to social conditioning (let's eat fast food), poor diet (more fast food) or too much money (put it on the plastic.)

Love

Hyper mania has different forms of affection.

In both cases you have to be trusted by the person. While a family context is very hard. Within a work context it is easier. Later we will talk about fools and relationships. Both are low contact for high periods of time, there is more compassion to the person and their physical and mental condition. Often they take a higher moral ground that other people. The stealth hyper maniac will see personal gain as a long experience, while the in-your-face will need to see a win in a short period of time.

To gain respect is harder with the stealth hyper maniac because while they appear relaxed on the outside, they trust very few people on the inside. However you can gain more respect with the in-your-face hyper maniac by conceding ground. Not seeing or hearing from either party is not a bad thing. Once respect is established, conversations are meaningful and secure unlike other groups where it's all false.

Both groups tend not to play with people's emotions. They can steer you in a direction, but often they are more willing to give you more rope to hang yourself. But only the stealth will nearly always pull you in.

They understand personal development; for those they trust they will let you make calculated mistakes. They debrief you on where it went wrong.

They might even put themselves up as a fool (discussed later) to learn more about you, your contacts or the way you work.

They love in a hands off manner, not saying words like I love you or having external affection. But rather knowing they have a person that cares for them, a good book to explore this is Cultures and Organisations [Author, publisher?]ISBN 1861975430.

Going nowhere?

You think your life is going nowhere?

Both groups do things for a reason. The stealth person would clean toilets or do manual work just to see how something works. These people do not fear death so the types of jobs they do could be dangerous.

Both groups like detail (to different extents) if they can't do it, they pass the job on to someone they can trust. You might not have seen someone with hyper mania for some time or heard their name in the news. Not because they have done things in a bad way but more because they are getting ready to move on.

Too much of one thing can spoil it. Jamie Oliver has been everywhere for six months. He needs to step out and come back.

In Hollywood there is a balance between stepping out and just not coming back. John Travolta was not main stream for twenty years, but when he came back he did it big style.

A hyper maniac will see opportunities, you might not hear of them but they are there in the background. There are times when a person can burn out or drop out (discussed later). They can bounce back or fall into depression.

Chameleons

It takes on average between 5 seconds and 30 minutes for a stealth hyper maniac to blend in.

An example of this was in Boston, USA when the passing traffic was asking **me** for directions. Blending in is what a stealth does best. Even within their own family they can often be invisible, because they can be. By blending in they get more information and can assimilate to the situation fast.

Only when the environment is mixed can you start to flush them out. Another example was in London at a Prize giving for the publishing awards. The people at the table I was on were so convinced that I owned a bank of magazines. They started to split the beans on circulation issues. The information gained quickly and moved a business on, when challenged about revenue streams a fully paid constant could not have done better.

The more often that they go out the better they are at cloaking themselves. Their highly retentive memory helps them to either feed back the same data in a different way or spin out a conversation that's a distraction away from them. Where they do not know the subject of conversation they intently study the person talking and learn from them.

The in-your-face sticks out like a sore thumb and if he is not centre of attention then something is up. He needs to be in the thick of things. He might not have attractive women around him but he will already know who is attending the venue and who he needs to talk to. He will not be blunt, because he knows how to keep relationships on the level. But if you are on his hit list watch out, he will extract all he needs.

During a recent trade show, a chap from India came on the stand with two others. He was dismissed by the owners but when after thirty seconds he said I want that product and further still kept on coming back. He was a wealth person with great ideas, but sold to as if a resident of Mumbai was selling to him, talking about dialects and areas along with the caste system. Only a stealth can do this effectively. His projects could increase the companies net profit ten fold.

Understand the people you are talking to, it does help.

The one to watch/sleight of hand

Both groups will use sleight of hand to different degrees. Some will say you are strategic, a key partner or important to the business. It's that NLP stuff again, others will love bomb you (spend so much time with you that you just can't think).

The only difference is the complexity of the tick. A good hyper maniac will split off the strong first and undermine them (not attack) in such a way that they have to follow, divide and conquer, the weaker ones will be forced to follow. These methods are covered later in Sun Tze and Genghis Khan.

The stealth hyper maniac will spend more time herding the cats (or people) into order, while the in-your-face will have two or three different candidates lined up.

A frequent trick used by the hyper maniacs is public confrontation in front of an office. Things like "you are with me, are you not, James?" Poor James can't get out of agreeing otherwise he will be ripped apart by the hyper maniac. Being put down by a hyper maniac is not good, even worst off he is an in-your-face type.

I have used sleight of hand many times. I was asked to evaluate a business by a friend and I realised that this was pyramid selling by the website. I decided to test the person (this is how hyper maniac let off steam, more later). The person called me on my mobile I said that I was on my way to a meeting on foot. They had 5 minutes, I really had 30 minutes. I asked what they know of my friend, they know only his name (great) and I then began to listen. He asked me what I thought of the online presentation. I said not "a lot", I then began to take full control the situation. This is when sales people lose control of the situation, when confronted by a hyper maniac. After 30 minutes not only did I have him agreeing that this business was unsuitable for my friend but also questioning what he was involved. Most of the time an in-your-face hyper maniac will control the conversation. This does not happen when a stealth hyper maniac wants something else. They control the format and direction, but not always the words.

Think of a hyper maniac's mind in the form of snooker. They know the outcome and objectives, they do not mind conceding red balls or other colours if they have to. But if they want they can (and do) score maximum break. How? They line up all the balls and are a few shots in front.

Think of a carpenter's mate, during the last few years before they go off on their own, a good one will be two steps ahead on the job. He will know how many screws to use; when to leave a section of glue to harden, and where to work next. He will be thinking on his own under the protection of the main carpenter. Once he has done this, he is ready to go out. If he goes out unprepared then his business will fail. Who invites a cowboy back to do bad work?

Hyper maniac plan, **boys do their plans**. The numbers of alternatives are also in their mind. They have five plans while a normal person has one. In a conversation they can take full control, answer questions before you think of them.

They are so flexible that they will keep you guessing. They often send fools off on wild goose chases. Or out to do their research because the fool is convinced it's a great idea. They are unlikely to get drunk or start a fight.

Time out

We all need time out. The in-your-face more than the stealth hyper maniac.

I have experienced in-your-face sales people fall apart. This chap, let's call him Lain, was on the top of his career (not his personal life) and had an income of over £150,000 plus expenses. I was known within his industry as an over achiever. Heaven help you if you stood in his way. I subsequently met two people that were pushed within three weeks of their first confrontation. Lain's issue was that he had bad personal relationship skills (a trait of in-your-face) and that you had to pay homage to him or he'd stabyou in the back.

Lain progressed from sales person to sales director, his personal turnover supported the company. The company grew and his income with it. However Lain became a victim. He was so in-your-face that one June he told the chairman "Give me any target - I will beat it". So the chairman did, he was after all riding on Lain's results. This was a bad time of year, fake jobs where booked in; the order book was full but the factory empty. By August there was no work in the factory and the work in progress showed a good month. Lain's reign was shattering to pieces, in September the factory moved and started with a clean sheet. There were now two directors: Lain and a chap called Don. Over the next six months Lain lost creditability with the board and ended up in the office for six months rather than gardening leave.

They needed to know where he was. His mental state was totally shot, one day he spent all day like a three- year old in a room with no TV or phone, banging a tube on the table.

His next role three months later was on a pittance of a salary, because the trade found out that he was let go for not achieving targets set.

Stealth hyper maniac are better off if they hit the bottom. They tend not to get depressed by working themselves up to a better position. They are more controllable of their emotions therefore and pick out a role that looks good on paper.

Would you rather employ someone that's been let go and had adverse press or someone with average results? The latter always wins until the former gets his house in order.

Back to NLP, the amount of time out positively is equal to the amount of control the person has on themselves. Therefore if a person of either type can control their emotions then they are more likely to have longevity of employment and stable relationships (more later).

Learning

A hyper maniac learns even while in a car, they use NLP.

NLP is all about programming your mind and the mind of others.

The hyper maniac, as stated earlier, is always a few steps ahead. They have a vision;, this must be how they do it! Sometimes it does not matter who gets in the way, sometimes they might be so ahead of the market it's a worry.

I picked up a report in September last year about e-books. They were soon to expand onto the global market, while they had been around for some years: the internet helped the sales.

I did my research over the following months and found out the market price and the suppliers of the service. The standard offering was restrictive so I made the product an easier offering.

After a one-hour presentation to the CEO, he allowed me to trail 5 books on Amazon and 20 on our own site. After five months the project was passed breakeven and 95% of sales are from the website not Amazon. The book trade even tries to order these books because their system does not know what they are.

You might learn but you have to apply it; see shoot the MBA.

Once you have mastered that NLP stuff, you can learn anywhere.

Hyper maniacs are very focused on reading. I only read book and papers that are targeted to my reading. Don't worry hyper maniacs like football rugby and other sports. They are very focused.

If a hyper maniac wants to know more about a business model or method of working, they will find out. They can gather information (as discussed already).

Fear & greed

Hyper maniacs know that fear and greed drive people. However they are not normally concerned about death, this makes them stronger.

For example, millions enter the lottery to win. However a hyper maniac knows that the odds are not in their favour. There are many scams on the net. The best ones offer 15% of someone's bank account. All you have to do is take the money into your account and then split it up. People are up for this, greed takes over all that all they can see is the money. The scam is to take an administration fee from you of £1,000 (Nigeria 317 letter scam), this scam is so bad in the UK SO19 has been set up to monitor it. [Not clear]There are 20 body bags sent back from the country that operate the scam every year. Don't worry on the other end the scammer is in fear of their life. If they miss the target they get a trip to the seaside (not nice) they are pushed off the cliff to the sharks.

Next time you see an e-mail from a man (or woman) offering you a slice of $50Million, you will know what they are trying to do.

At my brother's wedding his best man feared him because he had a water pistol filled with a liquid. He was in fear because he has always been in fear and not taken control.
The greed is something most sales people are told to use in presentations, however our hyper maniacs

use it to great effect. Both directly and indirectly, they will build up a database of greed or fear triggers.

For example I have met people that find being out of a relationship hard, they get off with someone just to be in a relationship. These people are easily corrupted into going off with the other sex, even if they do hate them.

Products are sold on fear and greed, look at Viagra, the fear of loosing someone, the greed of longer sex.

Fear and greed appeal to our animal instincts as well: the more controlled you are the less fear and greed control you.

A good hyper maniac (Stealth) will control themselves enough to say to an attractive person, "No, thank you, I am happily married." Or stay off drinking for long enough to learn from the drunken customers around them.

While the in-your-face will be up for both.

The less controlled a person is the more leverage you have with fear and greed.

Coming to terms with hyper mania

You can see that hyper mania is all around you. You might admit now that you are a hyper maniac or suspect a friend or relative.

We have covered many aspects of the condition; you need to start learning more about these people.

Coming to terms is easy, all you have to admit is that you are a hyper maniac. It's like having your first credit card. Do you use it carefully or do you blow it all?

The answer to that question is whether you are stealth or in-your-face. If you are in-your-face you will blow the lot, get leisure and enjoy. Stealth puts the card in a safe place after making a single transaction (small) just to test out how it works.

Now you are starting to get the picture we can move on to learning about NLP.

This is like your personal choke chain, you can learn to turn your emotions off. Once you have done this your will be very effective and dangerous.

Hyper mania in personal life

The history

I was born in 1960's into an advanced family, the fact that I was born in Newcastle does not bother me. It is in fact a conversation piece.

I consider my father a hyper maniac (of stealth) but as discussed earlier we all are a by product of our environment. My father has a very good business brain and questions most things. My mother is kind to others and within the community is renowned for helping out. I have two brothers and two sisters, all doing their own thing.

How lucky was I? In the 1970's our family holidays were to Spain (by car) in the 1980's they were to the Far East by plane. My parents wittingly or unwittingly were progressive and ahead of their time. By the age of 17 I had been to KL, Singapore, driven the Cameroon highlands. This was at the time when the masses were in Spain.

My parents' social network was very influential, as was their social status. However they cut me no slack. At the age of eleven pocket money from other activities was my money. They were not tight but careful.

I consider myself the hybrid of both my parents as to other degrees are my brother and sisters.

My childhood from five to eleven involved moving schools some five times. This was strange but I trusted my parents. The end result was to make me a more rounded person.

From the age of eleven, I attended a local secondary school. This was a social mix of working class to upper class. The school made this a level playing field. During this time (late 70's) there were a number of external issues, both before and after the Iron Lady.

At school I had a lowly existence keeping clear of the bullies, under achieving in results. I was bored not stimulated or challenged (but what's new) it was my extra-circular activities that I over indulged in, I found a niche to fill and fill it I did. This was the start of my road to stealth, but starting with more in-your-face.

By the time I had re sat my "o" levels I had won awards and had personal relationships with hundreds of my peers (more will be revealed about this and the exposure later). It did mean that at the tender age of nineteen, I went with a county high school for girls on their RE field trip. This consisted of 32 girls a teacher and parent, visiting 9 religions in a week. This opened me up to the power of the mind, NOT NLP I hear you cry!!! Yes six girls up all night in fear, two had a friendship bracelet that they could not take off.

I know what I have to do in life, I have known since I was sixteen. I amused people who ask me what I want for a birthday or Christmas. My response "world peace" because that's what I want. You can't take the world on its shoulders but you can take it into your heart. Like Bob Geldorf or Mother Teresa.

More recently I have been involved with charities in projects across Europe, talking to bank owners, finance providers and all sorts.

You can do it all with hyper mania

Just like PCP, you can with hyper mania. PCP or angel dust is sold in the USA. The police carry pump action shot guns because they shoot the limbs of people taking PCP. The super human strength comes from within, for stealth hyper maniacs and from the audience (or expected audience) for the in-your-face.

You could almost reprogram yourself, get control of your life and have everything your heart desires. If you are privileged enough to go to an Anthony Robins' conference you could walk on fire or snap wood with your hands.

Once you have set your mind and actions, the rest is easy.

It is that simple, positive mental attitude does it all. Strong will power is not to be underestimated, if you enjoy smoking and need to give it up then change the way you think about smoking. Instead of looking forward to a smoke think about a negative, the cost, the harm to your body or the fact that you smell like an ashtray. This mental thought will help your smoking decrease or stop, as you inhale the smoke you are filling your lungs up with tar, this mental picture will put you off smoking.

This is a simple form of NLP.

I have a direction, decide yours

As I have already stated, I know what I have to do, and I will. This is normal for a hyper maniac, but just the direction for stealth and in-your-face are different.

In sales, they are called hunters and farmers. The hunters go after the kill while the farmer grows his crop with loving care. In some cultures they are only hunters, if they have not had a kill for some time then the family could starve. Look at parts of Asia: they live off rice. There would not be enough meat to feed the population.

Planning your route is very important. While a journey starts with the first step, what if it's in the wrong direction? We plan to win, but some fail to plan. Stealth join up the dots in the plan created, while in-your-face take the direct route.

The book is full of personal experience and thoughts pulled in from being hyper maniac, yet also understanding the different flavours of hyper mania.

Now is a good time to reflect.

You can do a SWOT, or similar or just relax and think about what you have done and what you want to do.

The only thing holding YOU back is YOU.

You will always be

A hyper maniac, unless you use NLP to make yourself boring.

You see you might enjoy living on the edge or being behind some famous people. Or you might be the best sales person in the world.

You will always be:

- a son or daughter
- husband or wife
- father or mother
- worker or boss
- singer or dancer

but you will always be you

Think and question

Being a hyper maniac will teach you to question everything.

It is not dependant on which type you are but rather that it's in your programming. You will evaluate (or learn to) for yourself, yes, you will make mistakes but you are doing your own risk assessment of the situation.

For example, I was invited to join a company whose practices were just about legal, while the salary was great and the so called prospects good. They needed me more that I needed them, on the first interview they asked only about me, when I asked about the job, they simply said we will come back to that. I had done my homework and found out how they operated. After asking about the role, the office conditions more than four times. I said is it true that you're a life insurance broker? That you are looking for me to become an independent principle to sell polices to my network of contacts? The interviewer said no, we are a professional company operating in the insurance market. Anyway you appear not to be suitable. I found out later that it's not until the fifth interview they tell you about the company you see you have to be manageable (or gullible).

By doing your homework you decrease your exposure to adverse press. This is vital for the in-your-face sales person. It also means you hit the ground running, you know their markets, the company strengths and normally the office / company politics. We will cover this later.

You will also find this useful when going out to buy a house. Three years ago we wanted to move house. We went round with a clipboard, making notes on each property. We then used this data to make an offer; we knew from the data that the house might cost £200,000 but the repairs £50,000. Therefore the true cost was £250,000. We found a house where we knew what to expect.

This can also be applied to contacts you might have come across, what is their agenda? Why do they want a formal meeting? You will find that hyper maniacs hate time wasters and hate to waste time themselves.

An example is in one company I had worked in, sales meetings lasted 2 minutes per person plus 30 seconds at the end, they were run by an in-your-face hyper maniac. All the chap wanted to know was what you had achieved last week, what you expected to do this week. He would use double entry on a book and as long as the total figure was correct then he was happy. And if he was not he would give the group a mouthful.

An elephant is one big animal to eat, however you can eat him step by step. You set up phased objectives to reach, and reach them you do. And you will eat your elephant; it's traditional for the in-your-face sales person to be head hunted every 18 months (bad ones every 6 months). This means that they can either move on or stay and increase their salary.

While very good at their job, both types of hyper maniacs will leave employment in a creative way, thus letting the system work for them. I have booked a holiday for 14 days, then sent an e-mail to resign or given 2 days notice. Planning or timing is everything: the in-your-face sales person will move and take work with him; the stealth sales person takes the better customers and leaves a factory full of low margin high effort work.

The impact to the new business will be great, to the old business, hell.

You have to question everything:
- you
- your environment
- what you want out of life

THEN you have to do it, not plan, **do it.**

Stealth or Hyper Mania

As discussed already, with stealth it's timing and what you do not say. In a recent meeting I was not interested in what was being said, but rather the pecking order. This enabled me to go directly to the boss and focus my questions on him.

The conservative party campaign in 2005 was controlled by stealth, the number of seats reduced by employing the Australian election guru. His actions and his historic campaigns did make a difference.

Stealth hyper maniacs, like plants, hate staying in the spot light, they much prefer the shade. They are best at controlling the situation for someone else, they make exceptional mentors. I often get the 60 second call, it might be: we have been offered 50 free staff how can we use them? Or how can we increase our market share? They see things in shades of grey but also black and white.

A true example happened in March 2005 when I had a call from an IT specialist. He ready wanted to see how I was. He was concerned about his presentation on a multi-million pound install contact. The presentation was to a channel supplier, not the end customer. We discussed his proposition for 55 minutes and changed his presentation so much he rewrote it but won the business. For him the hardest part was overcoming payment. The example I gave was:

A man fills up his car with petrol; you are the petrol pump attendant (or cashier) and you have to make sure he pays for the goods. But how does he pay? Cash (because its burning a whole), credit card (because he has no cash), fuel card (it's not his car) or any number of other means. You see it's not up to you how he pays but rather that he does pay. You can't interface directly, your approach has to be compassion. You can help him by saying, that's 30 quid, do you have your credit card (assumptive close).

But when dealing with corporations that need products, they normally leave the payment to the FD, on the books, off the books, sales and lease back, sold to sister company or just pure cash. You need to understand your customer and their situation.

Wars are won by going out for it and by stealth. One only does not work but together the war will be won.

Life's rich tapestry

Why the hell do we do the things we do?

There are those that do what they want to and those that do what they have to. If you are a hyper maniac you do what you have to.

Because hyper maniacs are learning all the time, they are just like cows, they digest information four ways. They gather information and sort it or dump it. You might meet a hyper maniac and think, what a sad git. But when you need information who do you go to? That sad git or guru?

It lies in the rich tapestry because it makes a pattern and the pattern is there for a purpose. It shows the real you. Hyper maniacs, as discussed before, tend to use perception and reality rather well. There are ways to flush out the real them but if you look at what they have done and how they have done it, it shows their true colours. A word of warning is that hyper maniacs can tend to leave a number of contacts without knowing each other. They keep high level contacts together and these are not mixed with family members.

An example of an in-your-face hyper maniac gone wrong. This chap I spent nine months in a shared office with, was called Alistair. Both his business and personal life were a disaster. He had the gift of the gab and, selling a high value product, was a good salesman. However he knew nothing. He had to set up a different business every seven months because he spent all of the money. He left in his wake six investors nursing £200,000 in never-to-be-seen again investments (losses). His personal life was worse; when he got bored with a woman he left her and started with another. Four wedding cakes and seven kids later, he decided to settle down with a Russian girl, but little did he know: three years later she would leave him with her nice English passport. The picture he left was full of holes.

You might feel it's two steps forward and ten steps back, but life does that sometimes. You need to start with a good foundation.

Relationships

These are important in a person's life; no one likes to be left alone. If you are about to start relationships as a hyper maniac, choose a wife that understands, be faithful to her and you will have a solid foundation.

She will have a choice, steady (bad) income or the unexpected. If she can cope with the unexpected then you can't go too far wrong.

I have a loving caring wife, I spent ten years in a 24/7 environment. I could call up at 9 pm on Friday and say I will be back tomorrow. It's not that I was down the pub but rather that I was at work earning money. Most days I would get into work (not leave) by 7 am and leave by 7 pm (12-hour days), sometimes I would leave for work at 3 am, you see, hyper maniacs do not require too much sleep. Just drive to get the job done. This is one of the factors that make hyper maniacs different.

To take the pressure off my wife I bottle fed our children at 5 am, this meant they would sleep until 8 am and she would have a lie in. As they developed, they would not get respect until it was earned. We have one TV in our house, not because we are poor but rather to get three children to learn to agree. Attached to the TV is a PlayStation, Sky and a DVD. They have to agree (they are seven years apart) the play station has been taken away due to bad school results (up to five weeks) and has nearly been binned eight times in one year.

The Sky is only the basic package and has been turned off twice for three weeks. By only having one TV they have to communicate (including arguments) with each other. They do have toys in their bedroom. However they have a strict father and mother.

Other kids that come to our house have a TV in their room and a floor full of broken toys. I just follow the example of my upbringing. But when we go out I am often that proud of my kids, others I have seen are just animals. Some call it conditioning.

At the weekend we do Saturday and Sunday jobs, visiting relatives. My children know that they can't get out of this and they accept due to obligation and respect. There are plenty of children that have no respect for their parents or elders: this is bad.

Where they are family (or extended family) and you have no time for them, STAY away. I have no respect for my mother-in-law, in fact I call them the big kids (this is the way hyper maniacs ridicule people), they are worst than my 89-year old grand mother that we see on Sundays. They ring up because they have run out of milk, loo roll or need to talk to someone. They are a pain, when they once looked after my eight- year old I thought she was in charge.

As they say - if you want to be wise, stay with wise people.

The more you as a hyper maniac know about relationships, the more variety of relationships you have. The key ones are your family, they are your focus on earning income; love them or not they are your family.

The in-your-face or hypo maniac is less concerned about relationships. These are more deposable, he consumes people so fast he is onto the next before they know it.

The cut off

There are times when you need to walk away, not stealing any lines from Kenny Rogers and coward of the county.

As a stealth hyper maniac I can tell earlier than an in-your-face hyper maniac and they can tell way before the normal man when to walk away.

It's as much about walking away as it is the way in which you do it. The stealth hyper maniac would ask for further gathering time and information on a project (from him). The in-your-face hyper maniac would turn the meeting round to get an agreement to meet at a further date once they have come back to him (to him).

They are control related: the stealth that they appear in control, the in-your-face that he is in control.

They do not like burning bridges, but when they want to, they do more than burn them. I have seen in-your-face sales people physically destroy servers. Just to keep the company from keeping the data, or write to each client with a better proposal.

DO NOT piss a hyper maniac off. They are like elephants, they never forget.

Blending life

Hyper maniac home life is different to work life. Even the in-your-face hyper maniac does not want too much confrontation at home.

My children are great at misinformation, disinformation and deception. However they can't use it too often on each other because they can see it coming.

Having worked from home they do tend to pick up words or phases.

Being a hyper maniac is not all work, there is the fun aspect. You need to take time out and time with your family. You also need time away from the fools that surround you (to be discussed later).

Even a train does not go full speed all of the time; learn to take time out. You will find this a great period to learn

Ring fencing

As you grow older you will feel the need to ring fence relationships, not that you are hiding anything, but rather so you do not have to explain action to both parties.

Try not to be in someone else's pocket or you have a mutually exclusive life. This means you have a critic that might not understand your objectives or the bigger picture.

This is more familiar with women, but can happen with drinking partners.

By each group being exclusive you are not mixing family and work. My father was against me being involved in the family business and I am happy that I was not, I am my own man.

By ring fencing, you become a different person. I once worked in an open plan office and this chap called Jason was the hard man, he took no stick. He started up a relationship with a pretty young lady. However, the hard man dropped every time she called on his mobile. He became a sweet young sex kitten.

By ring fencing you are using your chameleon techniques.

Turning off

We all need to turn off and spend time with the ones we love or doing what we love. However an in-your-face hyper maniac can turn off more than a stealth hyper maniac.

If playing or looking at football, we need to get into the game, however hyper maniacs are good at duel tasking. They will let the brain work slowly through something subconsciously while the conscious is doing the activity.

The turning off is often considered as sport, however once you have been a hyper maniac you will find what it is. Normally for the stealth hyper maniac it's not drink, for the in-your-face it might well be drink. Find your ways of unwinding, this is key to relaxing.

The creator and founder of boo.com used extreme sport. He loved skiing (most in-your-face do), the fact that he concentrated on saving his skin meant that he could turn off from work.

There is often a band or track of music that might help; those calming music CDs are good for some. It might be a walk in the park or a power jog. Find out what it is and do it.
However it is not getting drunk, or sleeping around, or drugs. This is mind, body and soul unless you are a hypo maniac (in-your-face).

Cutting out

As already discussed, your environment feeds you. Most hyper maniacs tend to cut out coffee or caffeine-based dinks. They do have them when they need to.

They like to reduce fast food and prefer orange juice over fizzy drinks. They know that their body is their main tool for an income.

They also tend to have fewer days off sick because they eat healthier food, though they tend not to be vegans, just careful on what they eat. Many take trips to the gym or find ways of keeping fit.

Cutting out still refers to mind body and soul. I am happy to have given up drinking twenty odd years ago. Not that I do not want people to have a few drinks, but rather I am not worried about being stopped for drinking and driving. I do not wake up with a hangover. Too much of anything is bad for you, I will not waste four more trees with a chart. If you understand, then cut it out.

Your mind body and soul will improve as will your pocket. This amount of difference can really be surprising.

Do nothing to excess; too much of anything is bad for you. There are some vitamin C drinks that can change the colour of your skin if you have too much of them.

Kids

They are a by product of you!!! Only recently has Haynes, the car people, produced a manual for kids.

After the age of two the child will start to do what you do, they do it first to copy you. Then it will haunt you. It's all part of their environment and conditioning, they take both the good and bad. Beware they are a mini-you.

You have the God-like power to mould these offspring into a fully rounded person. You could also spoil their lives.

Some Hollywood types are either fully exposing their kids to their life style warts and all, others hide their family until sixteen or eighteen from the media.

The PlayStation generation can be multitask, from an early age they can start to process information faster. Looking at the game play, maps and figures at the same time. They use e-mail, MSN and iPods all at the same time.

This skill should be used to move things on. Start with Zoo Tycoon. This user friendly environment gives them money and animals. They will get a feel for marketing prices and business.

Then if you can build up to age of empires, age of mythology, strong hold and then Jurassic Park operation genesis. These games focus on evolving your culture and then the unexpected (loose animals).

Move up to Rome total war (£25 games £120 graphics card), this will teach them the type of troops and where to put them troops, and how to conquer.

By using these games in education rather than relaxing, you are starting to harden your kids. They have better dual processors, get them to apply what they have learnt.

My five-year old plays all of the above, does not understand most of it, but can play to a certain level. None are too blood thirsty, but reproduce culture and the make up of society.

Kids are familiar with queues. Go to any theme park and you think you are near the start. However you snake round and round until you reach the start of the queue.

While life is like this, it's just the perception that you are nearly there. This sense is increased as you can hear and see people enjoy themselves. Or a few minutes that you have been on the ride, you feel happy only to start the queue process all over again.

Where possible, take the kids aboard to learn a language or culture. This will round them off as a person. We are all stake holders in society.

You need however to balance what you have. The issue is that if your kid is a bright spark you need to help him at every step of the way. You can't give a man a net because then he eats all the fish. They must have a profiled education in progression; one year of good stuff followed by years of bad education can be to their detriment.

The under eighteens with skills after all are the ones that are creating computer virus, mobile phone viruses and havoc. They are bored: do something about it before they do.

Do a little at a time; blend it in with bringing them up.

Use this power carefully, it does come back and bite you.

Parents

Your parents have been and always will be your parents. Ok, you can do good or bad in their eyes, but they are still parents.

George W Bush and Barbara Bush must feel happy that their son is president. But he is still their son.

As a hyper maniac you are advised to hide what you do from these people Yes, they might understand but since they wiped your bottom, fed and clothed you, they still know best (they think).

If you are in the shit or need their help go to them, but I learnt from the age of sixteen they can be brutal and ask the most direct questions that cut through you.

My father was great. He would grill me about my next job, asking about the company, its funding, methods to market, market, my role and so forth. You knew when he was disappointed but also when he was happy. They do love you, they might not show it but they do.
This issue is best covered by Cultures and Organizations ISBN: 1861975430

I have learnt that families in business are bad, the first generation make it, and the second generation CAN (but might not) improve it. The third generation just piss it up again the wall. Two examples are the right way and the hell what happens to the business way.

The furniture company had been trading for 50 years, set up after the war it was a quality product made in the UK. Set up by two brothers it was a good company. By the time their two sons came to run the business it was still going strong. They had a passion for the business and were fundamentally good people. OK, they had flash cars, but their eye slipped off the ball. They had a board meeting and the CEO was not a man of action. They put the business up for sale and sold it.

The printing company, great company set up by a printer for his family, his son moved the business on into a new age. This son was respected by all who met him; no one had an unkind word: from the shop floor to the board, he had their respect. His son however bought in questionable business practices and surrounded himself with yes, men. He lost the company $30m over five years and no one liked him; he even created a coup to get on the board of the holding company.

While neither company was listed, what would you do?

Within society, your link with your parents is strong.

Extended family

My brothers and sisters are great; like my father I am very blunt with them. If I say no I mean no.

You should treat your extended family like your parents; keep what you are doing to yourself. You have very little to live up to in their eyes.

Worse still, they might not see the bigger picture. If you are the best employer in the town you will always get "Please employ Jimmy, he is a good worker". If they are so good at running business - let them do it.

These people can be bigger critics of YOU, even worse than your parents because they are jealous. They want what you have, if you are an in-your-face hyper maniac then they see the good car and the international travel, not the hard work.

I fortunately have very few of these, but to those who do, get it sorted.

These are the very people who can erode your mind. I once took my children to work. I showed them my office, then went downstairs and spent eight hours on a machine. The feedback to the extended family was that I had an office and that I did work.

75

This is why a hypo maniac (in-your-face) moves out of town, they can take risks in a different town and still return to their own.

Getting the balance right

While stress costs the UK £100Bn a year and 3 in 1 visits to the doctor are because of mental health: do not be a victim.

On a recent business trip, I met a very in tune person, who could see my mind racing but I still had my guard up. They spent three hours trying to understand me, however I was not prepared. NEVER share too much with a person at the first meeting.

Learn to get the balance right, if you are on a good income put up working with fools (discussed later). Then look to leave.

If you have issues with the family, then address them.

You might read a self help book, but without applying the subject you might as well have not read it.

By addressing the personal balances you will be a better person. Sure the hyper maniac has issues to address and address them they must.

At the age of seventeen I had a drink problem, I would go to the pub and drink as much as I could until the pub closed. At a party in six hours I drank a bottle of gin, a bottle of vodka and 16 cans of beer. I would have carried on but I was throwing up.

I realised the next day what a fun party and that I had a drink problem. I spent the next week on one drink when I went out then quit drinking - knowing that one pint would tip the balance to drinking again.

Do I miss it? No Hell. I do not waste money on drinks, if I am stopped by the police I know I can't lose my licence. My family knew that I stopped the next week and have not needed a drink since.
If I had carried on then I would have had a short life. It's now OK not to drink, but it was not twenty years ago.

Address the issue before it addresses you!!
These can be addressed via NLP.

Sleep

Like with many other things it's not the quantity but the quality. I know people that work a whole night shift and then sleep for only three hours.

Hyper maniacs tend to sleep for less than other people, they would prefer to work through an issue than sleep. 36- hour days are not unusual, in fact within the last fourteen years they are the norm.

If you consider, the financial markets open in the Far East on Monday and close in the USA on Friday. There is a maximum of two hours that the markets are not trading and you will find hyper maniacs can do this for years. They are great traders.

Once you get to grips with your hyper maniac you will become attuned to your bodily needs. The better the quality of food and sleep, the better the output.

Sex

Hyper maniacs have a better loving relationship; some in-your-face hyper maniac might prefer quick relationships. But it's almost by mutual consent. They are looking for a life companion. Even past relationships are more about caring than sex.

While for the in-your-face its more about conquest then move on.

Its not that they are unloving, more that they have an agenda.

Drugs

Stealth hyper maniacs tend to stay away from drugs, while in-your-face might use them for recreational purposes.

The fictional character Sherlock Holmes would have been a hyper maniac. When he got bored (unchallenged) he would resort to opium.

Steer clear of drugs, these include caffeine. You might use caffeine as I do to keep you awake when you need to.

However please note that most drugs have side effects or knock on effects. Take vitamin v, the drugs that help men perform better. There is talk that one could make you blind, the other lasts for 36 hours and can cause gangrene. Both have been sighted for increased sexual desire, which affects your relationships, which in turn affects everything else. Think of the poor woman who has to perform every night for four years. She shortly must get fed up after the first few months.

The other issue is that the amount taken increases to give the same buzz. Think about beer or wine, how much you had to take to get drunk. It increases as your body gets used to the dose.

By taking drugs only when you have to, in effect, makes your body better. How can you or your body perform if you have been on a bender all night? You and your body rely on each other.

Take it carefully, you need your body, the side effects of what you are taking, might come back to get you after many years.

Drugs are down to cause and effect.

Uppers and downers

As a hype maniac you will need to be able to change your moods just using the body's own chemicals.

OK so it's more NLP, no sweat. You can trigger happy, objective and sad conditions just by simple things like music.

A few years ago an army commander was fined for speeding. He was listening to music in his car, hears the charge and instinct told him to charge, he did so.

In the USA an army cadet was found guilty of shooting a group of people, before opening fire he had been conditioned to set off a whistle (which he did himself).

Watch your blood sugar level, this does drop like a stone with hyper maniac, you do not want to go hypoglycaemic.

You can push your body, but do not push it too hard. Find out what gets you down: it might be beer, night clubs or credit card bills and cut it out.

Push body and mind too much and they will get back at you. While for the in-your-face this is not an issue, as he is always moving on. For the stealth it's always a concern.

Great Hypo maniacs (in-your-face) have years of great work followed by years of depression. The hyper maniac is far more stable. It's just like the rabbit and hare.

Learn what makes you happy and conditions your mind to focus.

Love & marriage

To a hyper maniac love and trust are very similar.

Love is not instant, it can take time, however it can be over very quickly. Hyper maniacs tend not to show their real feelings. Only those close to the hyper maniac get to see the real person, expression of feeling.

Find someone who trusts YOU, I did, it counts.

Surely we have had our hard times, but the good ones have been great.

YOU have to ask them, would you prefer years of debt or the good life as we can afford it? If they really go for the latter then you COULD be Ok. Because while other people had flash cars my wife had a banger, but now she has a new car while others are worried about monthly payments.

To the in-your-face love and life are disposable. They move up and move on, often leaving a mess. This legacy does come back to find them.

Hyper mania in business

Unless you have a family pile, then you are in business for fun and for a living. Your business is YOU, not the products you handle or the deals you do, **it's you**.

People buy from people, they are buying from you. You might look good because your company or life style is flash, but they buy from you.

Business and family are best kept apart, let's get down to business.

Making a cup of tea is like business

A fool boils the kettle many times forgetting what he is doing.
In-your-face gets someone to do it, they always do it, but badly (getting your own back).
TQM, has spent the last 5 years studying tea and has an optima production.
Six sigma has the full flow production. [sorry not clear]
Six sigma plus, has water but only one tea bag left and that's for the wife. Without tea she is a bear with a sore head.

Building blocks

Everything you have learnt, directly or indirectly is a building block.

You might be young enough to remember your fist driving lesson, sat behind the wheel of a killing machine that also took you everywhere you wanted to go. As your lessons increased so did your skill until you did not stall the car or hit the kerb. You could multi task with your mind.

These are the building blocks.

Where you start building and what you are building with are also an issue to address. If you have good practical skills you do not want to be trapped in an office, if you have bad communication skills you do not want to start out as team leader.

I started out (with 5 O levels & 1 A level) selling chocolate, with a company. I was nineteen with a company car. Within nine months I would have been rep of the year.

You might have a bad environment, or be handicapped and reach this point sometime later in your life. It's not where you start as a hyper maniac but it's where you are going to. This subject is covered further later on in the book.

You build to your own pattern, because what you are building reflects you. What I am building I know in my mind.

Preparation

From building blocks you can prepare.

Once you have learnt to drive, you can prepare to go out into the big wide world. You need to plan where you are driving to who you are going to see. You will need fuel, if you do not have fuel your need is money. You might even need a present for the person you are seeing.

Proper **Planning** Prevents **Piss Poor** Performance: preparation is the key.

Like the journey, plan your life, not that you have your second child at thirty and your wife will be called Bo but outline what route you are looking to take. Just like the car journey there could be a detour, as a hyper maniac you need to take this in your stride.

Anyone that has seen a professional at work will see that he is prepared. He will have a van full of tools and gear. A cowboy will come round with just a hammer. If you have seen 'Toy Story' think of the professional that mends Woody. He has everything, even the kitchen sink. You need to be like this, as a professional: if someone asks a question you need to come back quickly.

The in-your-face hyper maniac would sometimes shoot from the hip, with the stealth would sound off real facts.

The hyper maniac creates the dotted pattern for his journey, the Hypo maniac goes hell for leather from A) to B) via the shortest route.

Plan, plan and plan again, beware plans change. But you won't, your route is set for your journeys.

Analyse not anulyse

Part of your journey will be analytical. In the car, on a motorway, you will need to judge when to pull out and when to stay in lane. But you can't afford to be overanalytical. If you do you could cause an accident.

You must look at the facts, decide what is of relevance, what information you require, what's not of use yet. You will need a good filing system in your brain and using paper.

Look before you leap.

Best described as:

In the local working men's pub two gents (not normally seen here) order beers and sit down. Two local builders are concerned about suited people in their pub.

When one suit goes to the loo, a builder follows him. At the wash basin the builder says "You look smart, what do you do?"

The chap in the suit says "I am a logical scientist."

The builder says "What's that?"

The suit says "I create logical patterns using facts. Let's give you a demo."

Builder says, "OK."

Suit says, "Do you have goldfish?"

Builder says, "Yes."

Suit says, "Pond or bowl?"

Builder says, "Pond, I built it myself."

Suit says, "The fact that you have a pond means you might have a big house."

Builder says, "Five bedrooms, built it myself."

Suit says, "Because you have five bedrooms, you might have children."

Builder says, " Yes, two lovely kids."

Suit says, " Because you have kids, you have an active sex life."

Builder, looking confused, still proudly says, "Yes."

Suit says ,"Finally, you have an active family life, have produced a house to live in, a family life with kids you love and have an active sex live. You are unlikely to masturbate."
Builder says, " No way, my sex is on tap."
They leave the loo and go back to their tables.

One suit turns to the other and says, "Type 45?"
The other says, "Yes, your round."

One builder says to the other, "You were there a long time, what did you find out?"

The one that had the demo said, "He is a scientist."

"A what?" he asked.

"Let me give you a demo?" he said.

"Ok, do you have goldfish?" he carried on.

The builder looked confused and replied "No."

"You're a wanker," his mate told him, "Your round then, wanker" he carried on.

The facts, the whole facts: that's what you need!!

Judging others

Try not to be too judgemental, because others will judge you.

Hyper maniacs do tend to keep their own council, more so the stealth hyper maniac than the in-your-face.

They know what goes around comes around; they are more likely to force someone to jump than push them.

It's correct that the first impression counts. I was nineteen and met a new area manager, some four years older than me. My first impression was not good, my old boss had a 2.3 litre car he had a 1.6 litre car. He dressed badly as if he was in the wrong role and ended up with no respect. At our sales meetings I had no respect for Jim and managed to turn his own team against him. He could not tell the regional manager because he would look like a fool.

It's not only you, it's others, the colour of your clothes is as key as the way you walk and the type of company you are in. For example if you are with a bunch of nerds you will not wear a suit; however bankers always wear pin strip suits.

Some born leaders can wear what they want because they are a born leader. People run them down because they are jealous rather than not liking what they wear.

And example:
USS Big Ship had her radar down and was heading to port.

"HMS Needle to USS Big Ship, 12 degrees to port."

"HMS Big Ship to HMS Needle, you move 13 degrees to port."

"HMS needle to USS Big Ship, you must move NOW or we will crash."

"USS Big Ship to HMS Needle, we are the world's biggest aircraft carrier, you move."

"HMS Needle to Big Ship, you move or you will crash, we are a light house."

Leaving a fool

In the kingdom of the blind the one-eyed man is the king.

There are plenty of fools around they will waste your time and send you on wild goose chases. Just steer clear of these fools.

I set up a team once, there were five people in this team and I made sure I knew each person's make up and thinking, how they worked and everything else. They left the company I worked for, to leave for the opposition. I kept in contact with them, they knew my clients, I knew theirs, they ended up stealing each other's clients. I kept mine.

If you have to deal with fools, keep your distance and evolve very little.

I once worked for a company that had a fool, he was the FD. Not because of his qualifications but because his family bought into the business. He gave me a verbal warning for installing software on my PC. I told him that I would not remove it but let the IT director remove it. A week after being told off, he came to me because he needed to use this software. Try not to play a fool at their own game, you do not need to come down to that level, rather keep your distance.

Shoot the mentor

Many people have need of a mentor; Anthony Robins' mentor is a great number of people. The role of the mentor is to help the situation by discussing the issues of the day, in that person's life, give them direction. I have nothing against the few good mentors. I do have an axe to grind for the mentors that destroy hope.

However over the last two years, the co-founder of Chipmunka Publishing has been offered mentoring services. Some of these people should be shot. They are offering high level solutions where the issue is that someone needs to get the work done. Living in the clouds does not pay the bills.

They like that the consultant will come in with your business situation resolved in their mind. Remember you could (and hyper maniacs are often) better than them. Ask for references first, make sure that they have helped others. Talk to them first on the phone.

I know people that expect results from these people, they need to prove they are good to you. You might need to mentor them. One mentor once offered to change the model of the company that I was involved in: to decrease the amount of admin he recommended putting everything on line via a retailer. I managed to convince the CEO, that this was not best for the business because our GP was 50%. That would reduce it to 20% and out on costs [not clear]would be the same. The person concerned did not understand the business. One size does not fit all.

To my horror, at a meeting in London, a mentor broker was trying to sell his services. While the candidates did not have experience in our sector, he charged £700 per introduction. We asked for a role and gave a job description; he was unable to fulfil the role.

If you need a mentor (or feel you do) they should be recommended to you and you should feel equal to them.

If you are jack of all trades and master of none, be a mentor.

Shoot the MBA

In the ideal lab, we have control. In the real world it's hell. Most, but not all MBAs live in a sterile world where cause and effect are linear (2D), while life is 3D.

Being an MBA along does not prove anything, being a CEO of a good company and an MBA is different. You only have the MBA, after you have proved yourself.

I admire few MBA's, I admire many people that are making an impact in the world. If Richard Branson studied an MBA would it make him any better? Or if you bought one from the University of South Hampstead.

There are those MBA's that are so good, it's great, there are those who have had to do it because they can't get a job. I spent sometime with a couple of MBA's and was not impressed, while others I have met I have great regard for.

If you are a poor MBA, you will find the tools area helpful.

If not, do you know:

- how to set up a limited company in your country on line?
- where to get audited accounts

- where to buy websites
- which type of bank account to have
- how to create money in a business
- why you take the kitchen sink to all investors meetings
- why not to use the larger firms
- do not pay the upfront fee
- why you do not have to have the property with the business
- when to walk away
- when to roll up your sleeves

If you do not be a constant or mentor, otherwise LEARN from the **tools section [not clear]**

Shoot the consultant

As the consultants teach the trainees: give a man a fish and you can give him another tomorrow, give a man a net and he does not need you.

A great example is:
In our days awash with consultants this should make many of you smile.

The Yuppie and the Shepherd: A Modern Day Parable

A shepherd was herding his flock in a remote pasture, when suddenly a BMW charged towards him in a cloud of dust. The driver, a young man in a Prada suit, Gucci shoes, Dior sunglasses and a D&G tie, leans out the window and asks the shepherd: "If I tell you exactly how many sheep you have in your flock, will you give me one?"

The shepherd looks at the man, obviously a yuppie, then looks at his peacefully grazing flock, spread out over an entire pasture and calmly answers, "Sure --- why not?"

The yuppie parks his car, whips out his Dell laptop, connects it to his AT&T mobile phone and surfs to a NASA page on the internet, where he calls up a GPS satellite navigation system to get an exact fix on his location, which he then feeds to another NASA satellite that scans the area in an ultra-high-resolution photo.

The young man then opens the digital photo in Adobe Photoshop and exports it to an image processing facility in Hamburg, Germany.
Within seconds, he receives an e-mail on his Palm Pilot that the image has been processed and the data stored. He then accesses a MS-SQL database through an ODBC connected Excel spreadsheet with hundreds of complex formulae.

He uploads all of this data via an e-mail on his Blackberry and, after a few minutes, receives a response. Finally, he prints out a full-colour, 150-page report on his hi-tech, miniaturised HP LaserJet printer, turns to the shepherd and says: "You have exactly 1,586 sheep".

"That's interesting. Well, I guess you want one of my sheep," says the shepherd. He watches the young man select one of the animals and looks on amused as the young man stuffs it into the trunk of his car. As he is ready to drive off, the shepherd says, "Hey, if I can tell you exactly what your business is, will you give me back my animal?"

The young man thinks about it for a second and then says: "Okay, why not?"

"You're a consultant," says the shepherd.

"Wow! That's correct," says the yuppie. "But how did you guess that?"

"No guessing required," answers the shepherd. "You showed up here even though nobody called you --- you want to get paid for an answer I already knew --- to a question I never asked --- and you know nothing about my business. Now give me back my **dog**. The number quoted was based on my uncle's flock not mine and you pulled this stunt this morning on him."

The consultant knew nothing, even less than what he had in his hand. The report offered was not only incorrect but second hand.

They get **you** to rely on them but they are more dependant on **you**. But they can't let **you** know that their fat salaries are from you.

Look at the top four accounting firms in the 1990's. The audit of accounts was perhaps 20% of the fees. All capped and to a price, while the constancy was 80% of turn over high margin and easy.

You can't ask for a reference from these people. How could you say? "Tom is a creative chap, we enjoyed giving him £200,000 to tell us we were bust. I then sold my house because the bank told me to."

One company that I have met had a turnover of £35,000,000. They injected £400,000 into the company from its parents just to keep it going. The bank insisted on a full report, costing the company £40,000. All the bank read was the summary: liquidate.

Most consultants I have met, like meetings or even better, meetings about meetings. They really like meetings about meetings, about something that can't happen, in a hotel in the sun on someone's expenses. Because they are so high level, anything they want can't happen.

Some of them are to be trusted, but these are not as obvious as not parking the horse out the front. Make sure that they have a passion for your project, double question everything.

I attended a product launch for consultants on HMS Belfast. I sat back and enjoyed the fun,;they could not see anything other than their next assignment. I was lucky to meet a chap call Eric (he had a brain). While the others talked about 4-month contracts I explained mine were decided in the first 30 seconds. If they could not or would not change to save their company, I was out. Over 95% stated that they would stay for the fee, not me, I had standards. But they could not see this.

I pointed out how and why the food was presented the way it was. **Most could not get it, but that's consultants for you.**

What comes first

I have had three years of pain. I have burnt a heap of cash and have 243 product lines to bring to the UK, with a total turn over of £100m PA. If I had bought a company in the first place I would not have had the time to find these products.

This in most terms is considered, the front (business) or back office (admin & support). I have come to realise that the front office needs to be equal to the back office, however without effective back office (see six sigma) [what does this mean?]you could lose money without knowing it.

Good front office, we were trying to save a business. The sales director was a head of target. The company was happy, however they had no product to sell as it was all made in China. Some of it had not been made.

You might be the best sales person in the world but without product you have no income or credibility.

Good back office. A dynamic company burnt £120,000 in marketing material for its oil portraits, they had great pens, marketing material and web site. The ordering system was very high tech. However their only sales person was the CEO. He was considered by most prospects mad. They did not close any business.

You need to do both, production (or admin) need to feel equal to each other. Then the company will grow. Imbalance creates a loss in both money and staff.

Again it's all down to balance, if it's your money then you need to spend it wisely. Add 10% for over runs, keep the costs under control.

If you are into production, find a salesman (you can trust), if you are a salesperson find someone good at production and costs.

There is a real need to have a system in place when you get an order and a person getting the orders.

You might have the best website, with fully integrated SQL, but if no one uses it then what's the point? While if your site is out of date then your shipment might be going out late or the whole business costing you too much.

You and your business need to evolve, but you need to start somewhere. This is called a **vehicle**. The company used to start the ball rolling.

Six sigma

Six sigma is a principle used to increase productivity in a controlled fashion. There are comities, however when done properly and focused it can produce great results.

Six sigma sits alongside good management, they will apply some principles but not the whole process.

An example of a company, not using six sigma is:

a flat pack company in Rotherham, UK, with a turn over of £35m. It called in the receivers, upon investigation has had one production mess and one sales mess. The production was fundamental, it produced what it wanted, not what the customer wanted. This led to £1m of stock that was over two years old. The sales mess occurred as it only had three customers, because it did not understand sales. Over the year before it stopped trading the production included a number of 750 ranges; in the last few months it was down to 250. These were not high volumes. The directors took out bank loans and started the factory again. In 2005, one of these customers stopped buying flat pack.

An example of six sigma:

an auto motive manufacturer had 37 nuts and bolts on its car. They had 5 shut downs a year and 5 suppliers. They now use 4 nuts and bolts, one supplier, with one as back up. They are more productive, better after sales and more profitable.

Therefore six sigma is designed to make the operation faster and better. Like anything it must be implemented well.

A great book to lean more is 'The Six Sigma Way [author? Publisher?]isbn 0071358064

Six sigma plus

Six sigma plus is following on from six sigma looking upstream and downstream for issues.

An example is this: you might be a manufacturer of tyres. thinking about your new range, should it be up market or down market?

If there is a shortage of rubber, the prices will increase by 30% therefore you need to be in the premium market to protect yourself.

If you do not use six sigma, do use six sigma plus. It will have a far bigger impact on your market.

Everything is becoming a commodity, German farmers are being made bankrupt by cheap under priced milk in the shops. You will find as discussed already that raw material prices like oil price are increased. This increases the prices of the product, decreases your margin.

Tesco in the UK have created product deflation over the last 10 years. Jeans are £4, trainers £5 and electrical products cheaper than anywhere else. The only issue is that these products are unbranded, they are made in the same or similar factories. Rather than dealing with product brokers, Tesco are big enough to deal with the factory direct.

Swot

Any business book will teach you about SWOT.
Strength, weakness, opportunity and threat.

However you can justify most business decisions
using a tainted version of swot. There is no
correlation or rating in your swot.

A typical chart looks like this:

S.W.O.T.

STRENGHTS:	WEAKNESSES:

THREATS	OPPORTUNITIES

A good step to this first approach is to S.W.O.T. ourselves:

DON'T PANIC!

It has to be laid out accordingly, please do this on paper and be real with yourself:

FILL IT IN, Think about IT

DO IT

<u>UNDERSTAND</u>

STRENGTHS:

- Knowledge & Expertise
- Establishment
- Product Quality
- Product Definition
- Service & Accessories
- Image
- Pricing Policy
- Customer Focus
- Planning

OPPORTUNITIES

- Government Legislation
- Industry Standards
- Monopolies
- Market Niches
- Changes in Customer Attitudes
- Exports
- New Technology

WEAKNESSES

- Manpower Resources
- Financial Resources
- Knowledge & Expertise
- Lack of Customer Focus
- Product Orientated
- Pricing Policy
- Image
- Sales/After Sales

THREATS

- Government Legislation
- Industry Codes of Conduct
- Barriers to Entry
- Price Wars
- Changes in Customer Attitudes
- Imports
- New Technology

Now do Competitors S.W.O.T.

Competitor 1

Competitor 2

What do you and your business have going for you? What does the competition have going for them?

A hyper maniac will challenge each entry, give them a weighting and then apply a formula: $S + O - W + T = result$. This gives a clear picture if the hyper maniac needs to proceed.

Try it and you will be amazed at the results. Justify your actions by fact rather than emotion. If the cars are the same price, but one has better MPG lower cost of ownership but a Skoda badge, you will go for the nice new Ford.

Your SWOT is overridden by emotion.

Example:

A chap has an arranged marriage: he can choose one of three girls. Mary is a size 8 careful with her money and has own flat. Louise is size 12, good job, flash car and lives at home. Emily is size 20, a lawyer and earns over $1,000,000 a year.

Which does he go for? The one with the big tits (emotion).

Streamlining

Streamlining any business creates and loses jobs, money and futures.

Everything runs in cycles; the 2005 objective is to outsource everything. This increases return on investment for your investor. Yes, you might lose control, but it's all the fashion.

There are some companies like Dell, Cisco and others using this process, along with e-commerce lead solutions that become faceless and simple to use. Anyone who has used DHL or UPS, will love the online shipping. You can track the parcel in real time, the cost to the business has been great but the number of calls asking where the packet is and who signed for it reduced.

The business does benefit from this type of transactions however it all depends on your partners, you need to trust them.

A real example is the automotive industry, they use just in time, streamlining and pen book like this:

The production cycle for a mass market car is held in the main frame, all suppliers can see this data. Let's say that the car needs alloy wheels and leather seats. These are subcontracted from a supplier, they know that the green seats are required at 10 am and they will be fitted at 11 am. The contract they have is one hour before, this means delivery is at 9am. There are financial penalties if they do not get it there on time, but by using these methods, they offer effective production. The auto manufacturer can raise billing for them too.

The margin might not be high but the business is so streamlined that it is great.

Ford and other automotive manufacturers try and reduce costs by 5% a year and they can do this by using common parts.

The easiest way of understanding common parts is in fast food.

The burger house only has 67 raw products in its bill of materials, 4oz burger, 8oz burger, cheese, sauce, big buns, small buns, burger boxes and salad. There are three sizes of cup and six syrups. However they can produce many different flavours and toppings.

It's not what you have got; it's what you do with it.

The downfall of streamlining can be demarcation. If it's not in the contract I am not doing it. In-house teams will understand the common good, others will refer to the contract. This is the difference in partner!!

Fiscal 2

Do not believe the accounts. Because you have a clean driving licence does not mean that you have not been stopped for drinking and driving.

The accounts of a company can be 18 months out of date, in the case of Parmalat, Enron and others they could be wrong. While they give you a good snapshot of the company, there are issues that need addressing.

Most companies using the new accounts standards are bust. Many are cash cows, producing cash before it's due on small margins (supermarkets); the balance sheet looks good but the business is not. Others are geared rather too heavily. If a company has millions of assets and the bank won't lend it further funds, does that not say something?

Read the bluffers' guide to accounting, this will get you on the right track. The accountants are there for a role, it's not in your interest to find out what that role is.

The new accounting standards will make it clearer who has no money and who to invest in. But watch out for things off the books …

Understanding your limitations

Inspirational quote
Know your enemy and know yourself
Sun Tzu, The Art of War

If you can't do it, you can't. You might want to learn.

I recently have to move a site to PHP for a company. While I understand HTML, java and JavaScript I know nothing about SQL and PHP.

I did something wrong and told the IT chap, I do not know what I am doing, I can't fly a plane, do brain surgery or repair an engine. If I do it wrong again it's because I do not know what I am doing.

There are some things you just can't do, there are others where you learn to do them. There are yet more where you just do not want to do them.

Before PCs were mainstream, I worked for a company who every day had to interface with the main frame. After four weeks I ended up doing it, I did not enjoy it. So I did it wrong one day and was banded by the boss from doing it. Everyone but him knew that I wanted to move on and I did.

There are times when you need not get your hands dirty, just move on to the bigger picture. While there are others when you need to prove you can do it.

There might be times when you want to see how others could do it.

Know your limitations and stick to what you know. Hypo maniac tend to spoil things that they do not know.

Boo.com

Do read the book, you will see a company who had it all, yet had nothing.

There are businesses I have invested in that have been before or after the crest of the wave. You must consider this opportunity and if it will do what is says on the tin.

By offering a better product for less money or more effective solutions is that going to in? {Not clear]

Boo.com had the back end sorted at a cost, but the front end just was not there. They had investors to worry about. They needed money like it was going out of fashion.

The final resolve was not the best. Just be careful, others judge you by your failure. It's better not to back a horse than to back a loser.

There are many examples of markets moving to keep the investor out. The stock market is the ideal one, it goes up and down. For some periods it might trade sideways.

People in the UK were piling into buy-to-let after the party had finished, do your own homework. You will win more than you lose.

You fail your first five businesses to succeed in others.

Learning to walk away

This is a continuation of the previous subject. If it is not for you, walk away.

They might be fair or only ask for £10,000 but after doing your homework if it does not add up walk away.

I have already told you about the job that was wrong. But there are not only jobs but also companies.

Would you buy a house if it was valued at £300,000 with a monthly repayment of £1500 and rental income of £2000? That's what they told you, but the difference between perception and real kick in, the small print said that this rental was for 6 months; thereafter it was at the market rate (£600). What would you do now?

Yes, I have bought houses and land without seeing them, but I did my homework.

Often you can't even talk to the people, just distance yourself from them, that's all you can do.

The 80/20 rule

80% of effort produces 20% of the result. And it does.

You might have a client list: the ones where they need to have their hands held are taking up your time and only producing 20% results. The ones who come in and out are the ones you need.

By focusing on who creates more margin, not turnover for you or your business, you can create more value. Increased value means increased worth.

Increased turnover could lead to increased work and very little return.

Reduce your interaction with time wasters think smart.[unclear]

Winning

You are a winner, you will win:

whatever the battle you aim to win. The methods have partly been discussed in Genghis Khan and Sun Tzu.

No matter what you do aim to win, an easier way of doing this is have good team players. While they might not get on with each other in times of trouble they can cover each other.

Winning is to think of what you do in every day life, just by taking part you might be winning. Each day has its battle, win the battle and win the war.

You are a winner, you will win.

Playing the fool

The fool or patsy should be avoided; you do not want to be like them. However, sometimes you have to play the fool.

Once on a business trip, I was in the company of an in-your-face sales person. He was not a hyper maniac, just a salesman. Since I was to present to an overseas lender I needed him on my side. Therefore I played the fool to him and I waited for every word (or so he thought), I was the lap dog. However I needed this contact, I needed the funds for my project but I also needed to know how this chap worked.

We spent four days together and I just let him talk. While I could not take him head on, I could start to question some of his statements.

By day two, I had what I came for, the offer on funding. Therefore I needed to work on this chap. The more I questioned, the more he gave out and guess what, 80% were lies. At a debriefing to a team member, who was keen to offer his projects to the lender. I proved that what had been told in the UK was not true and could not be done. All of the information extracted from the chap was used as proof.

Fools are easy to spot. Look at the news, there is someone reading a statement, they do not know the situation; they are just there to present the statement. The people behind the action want to stay out of the firing line.

Keep your friends close, but your enemies closer still.

The truth about money

Money is useful. However, the love of money is the root of all evil.

Money is also a state of Mind, *Think And Grow Rich* is a good book.

This is true. As greed takes over, there are people left behind. I am not saying you should sell all you have, but rather be careful with money. You will need to borrow it and pay it back.

Since the enterprise act of September 2004, people and companies in the UK have become more flexible in their understanding of money. However banks and lenders do not like risk. The bad debit (not performing loans) in Japan is so vast that the numbers are scary.

Just by playing a simple game of monopoly you can find out how people are with money. Do you buy no houses and the money runs out towards the tail end of the game? Do you buy all the property that you land on and become asset rich cash poor? Or are you in the middle?

It's very easy to spend money, harder still to save it.

Sun tzu

The art of war is such an inspiration. However it was designed to be a practical instruction in life and war.

However most people use this book as a coffee table book or to add to their CV as last book read.

It is a practical book, my son who plays Rome Total War is reading it (aged 12), not for a good read but for a good battle.

Why do people buy presents like cookbooks? Because the receiver is crap at cooking? Why do people buy their contacts many gifts? To highlight in a non- verbal way where they need to improve.

Sun Tzu covers battles, while the principles are similar, he covers battles. The theory is still being used by Sandhurst and other army training institutions. But furthermore they are applying the principle.

Why have a book in French if you have not read it or the complete collection of Shakespeare still in the box?

We are here to live and learn, hence the author only reads in a focused fashion.

Genghis Khan

What a man! He concluded internal conflict before resolving external conflict.

Yes, he did kill many of his own countrymen, but it was kill or be killed. He had a system that worked, he would offer peace and if not taken, there would be blood shed. The stories of his tribe doing everything on their horses are true. To bring the tribe into line, he would kill those that did not stand with him, leaving only those under two feet to be added to the extended tribe. Once he was king, he picked out other countries but he used stealth.

He would go to a board [unclear] town, seek peace (or occupation). If they did not agree he would kill them all, except the scribes. They would be set free to tell the next town what was coming (viral marketing). He would use the towns' own animals to stamp [unclear]the towns, he would use people in cities.

He adapted and became better, understood trade between conquering cultures. He would use daring to attack forces. He would promote people that had skills. They need not be from his tribe, he could trust them.

What has this got to do with businesses?

He forced the competition out of the market. Shut off supplies, created fear, viral marketing, free trade and learned how other people work.

The tools of the trade

This is the rub, if you have seen these and understand how and when to apply the information, it's a refresher. If you have seen these and still don't understand try again from the start!!

If not - do you know:

- how to set up a Ltd company in your country online?

For the UK you can use www.uk-plc.net
For the USA you can use
- the internet to compare prices on a state by state basis

For the UK you need to use
www.**companieshouse**.gov.uk/
- Other charge over this amount for a different service.

For the UK you need to use www.reg-123.co.uk
For the USA you can use www.reg-123.co.uk

- Which type of bank account to have

A business account fool, [unclear] keep business in a different bank to your personal
- How to create money in a business

Factoring, AR, CID. Trade finance and overdraft should all be familiar to you
- Why you take the kitchen sink to all investors meetings

If you know the in and out of a proposition then they will feel comfortable and better still if you take the contract sign, you are for real
- Why not to use the larger firms

Unless you want PI, cover a smaller firm. It will be more flexible and cost less

- No to pay the upfront fee

Advanced fee fraud is great fun, do not do it.
Unless you want to lose money

- Why you do not have to have the property with the business

The property will increase the amount you put into the business and change the way you operate

- When to walk away

If you can't afford it, walk away

- When to roll up your sleeves

Workers get things done, lead from the front

What do you know?

If you learn nothing, then how is life cleaning up?

You have to learn, there are few jobs for life. This section of tools is just to keep you going. It's practical if you use it and if you don't, then sorry you are bored.

The publisher is upset because of the amount of space used, but you are going to fill this section in.

Worse still you are going to use the information supplied (by you) to think about what you have to do.

It's OK, 80% of you who apply yourselves will still be in the same job, just have spark. 20% will have realised that they need to move on, soon but not now.

You are holding yourself back. The rest is an excuse, because your feet are under the table and you are comfortable. I am sorry if this section upsets you and your business, but this book probably will.

Use a pencil, think, but do it.

1.1 S.W.O.T.

| STRENGHTS: | WEAKNESSES: |

| THREATS | OPPORTUNITIES |

1.2 My business's products and their respective contribution to turnover:

Date _____

	Current year %	Last year %	Previous year %

Observations:

1.3 My business's customers and their respective contribution to turnover:

Date _____

	Current year %	Last year %	Previous year %

Observations:

Appraising the market

2.1 Understanding our position

DON'T PANIC! Do it again right!! Measure twice, cut once.

S.W.O.T. stands for Strengths, Weaknesses, Opportunities and Threats and is laid out correctly:

STRENGTHS:

- Knowledge & Expertise
- Establishment
- Product Quality
- Product Definition
- Service & Accessories
- Image
- Pricing Policy
- Customer Focus
- Planning

WEAKNESSES	
• Manpower Resources • Financial Resources • Knowledge & Expertise • Lack of Customer Focus • Product Orientated • Pricing Policy • Image • Sales/After Sales Support • Planning	
THREATS	
• Government Legislation • Industry Codes of Conduct • Barriers to Entry • Price Wars • Changes in Customer Attitudes • Imports	

2.2 Product/customer matrix

	Star:	Question mark:
HIGH		
LOW	Cash cow:	Dog:
	LOW	HIGH

MARKET GROWTH RATE

MARKET SHARE

What are you doing to do about your:

Stars:

Question marks:

Cash cow:

Dogs:

2.3 Competitors S.W.O.T.

	Key Strengths	Key Weaknesses

Competitor 1

Competitor 2

Competitor 3

3.1 Customers and consumers for my organisation

PRODUCT	CUSTOMER	CONSUMER

4.1 The product life cycle

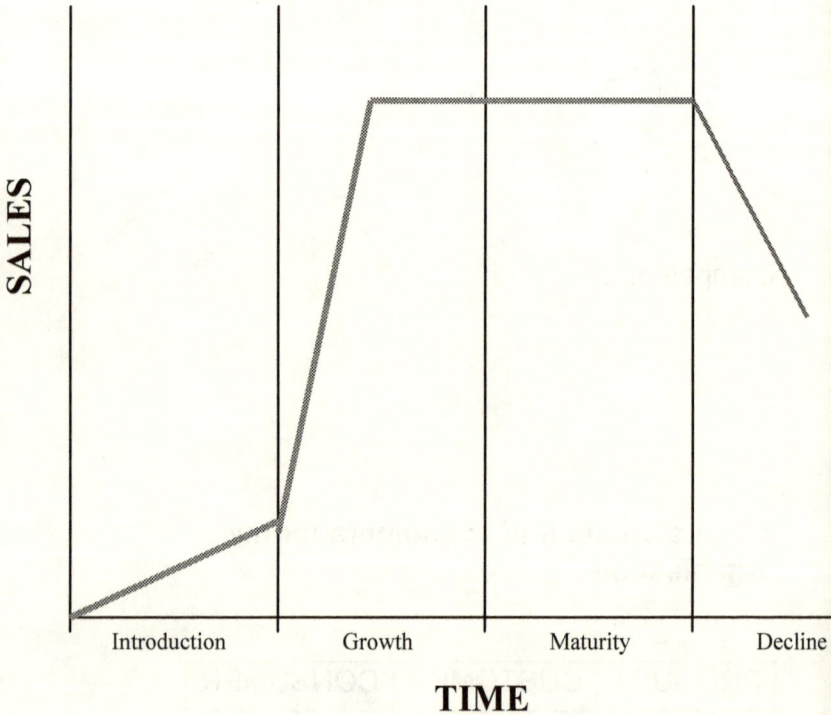

A graph with SALES on the vertical axis and TIME on the horizontal axis, divided into four stages: Introduction, Growth, Maturity, and Decline.

How are you going to ensure that products in the introductory and growth stages achieve their full market potential?

What are your plans for developing or replacing products in maturity or decline?

Do you care? What is the purpose of the company?

5.1 Promotional techniques my business could use to pull customers through the AIDA:

AWARENES

INTEREST

DESIRE

ACTION

5.2 Appropriate media for my business

List them you might only need three types

5.3 Appropriate stories for the media

Suitable stories that have occurred in the last 12 months:

PRODUCTS
MARKETS
PEOPLE
POLICIES

6.1 Features Vs benefits

Features that my Business offers	Benefits and Importance to the Customer

7.1 Business & Marketing planning

1. What does this Business actually do?

2. Is it doing what was intended?

Yes: ☐   How?
            Why t? [unclear]

NO: ☐   How?
           Why not?

3. What should it be doing?

4. How should it be doing it?

7.2 Understanding the Process

SET UP TIME

A machine tooling company uses a variety of metal thicknesses. They assume that the greater the metal thickness, the longer the set up time. However they have never established this and so have failed to identify the true relationship between these two variables.

By logging the set up times against the different thicknesses and then plotting them accordingly, the company can see how close the relationship between metal thickness and their respective set up times is.

PARETO ANALYSIS

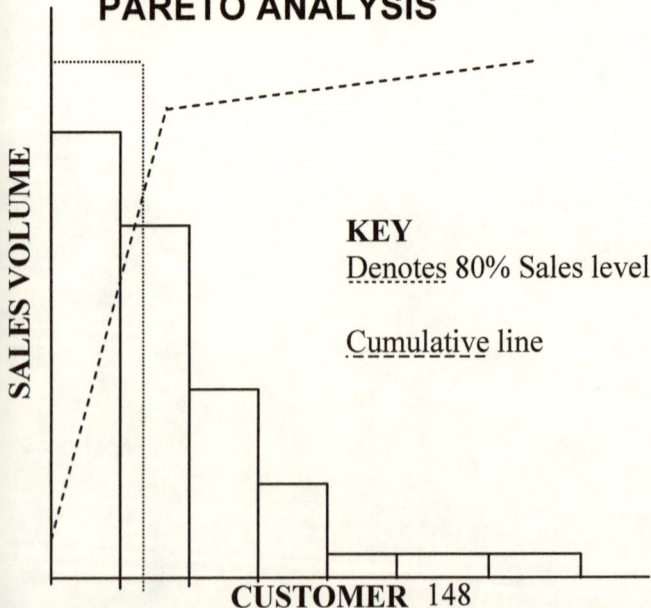

KEY
Denotes 80% Sales level

Cumulative line

The graph illustrates the 80:20 ratio, so often experienced in business situations.

In this particular situation, we see how 80% of sales come from 20% of customers.

CONCENTRATION DIAGRAMS

In 1854 Dr. Snow used a Concentration Diagram to identify that a large number of victims of the cholera epidemic were from Broad Street.

This enabled him to realise that all the victims had used the same water pump.

He remedied the situation by closing the pump.

Carnaby St. X	Beak St. x
Lexington St. x	Poland St. x x

Malborough St.	Broad St.
	   x x x
	  x x x x

8.2 Marketing plan

Objective: -

Appraisal: -

Strategy

Product: -

Placement: -

Price: -

Promotion:-

Finance: Key Comments: -

Opportunities:-

Risks: -

Timetable: -

Source of information

Highlight some key sources of
information that may be used to help
improve knowledge of a new market and
customer area.

You look at your client base; they will
give you a clue, by market and by
product.

To build an outline of the industry
This is useful to include within the Business Plan, to
demonstrate how the intended development of the
company relates to the development of the industry
as a whole. In particular it gives added strength to
the report when it is being examined by third parties
such as the Bank.

Items that should feature within the industry outline
are:
- Summary of major activities within the
  industry
- Indication of industry growth rate
- Appraisal of who is being
  successful/unsuccessful and why?
- Primary identification of niches not being
  satisfied within the industry

BAR GRAPH

SALES	AGE
100	16-29
300	30-44
200	45+

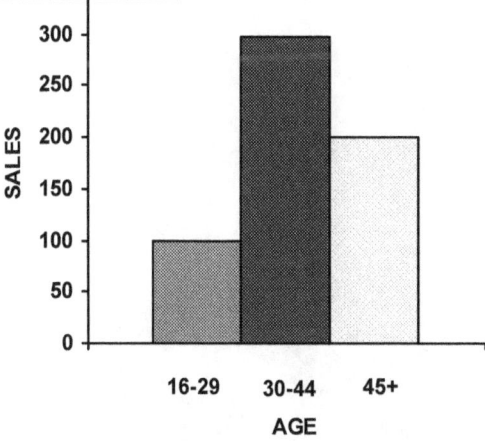

PIE CHART

MARKET SHARE %	COMPETITOR
40	X
30	Y
30	z

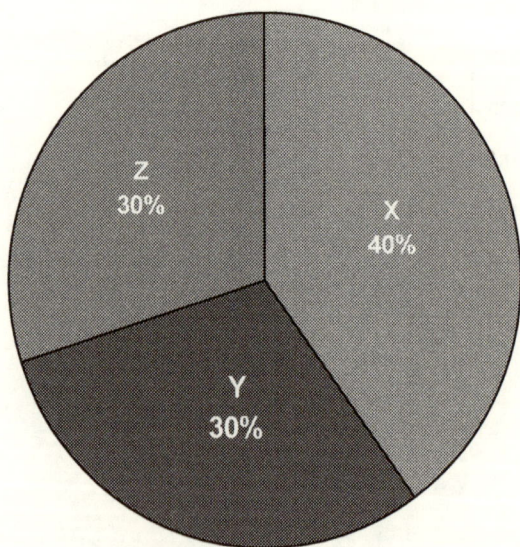

9. Attending an Exhibition

9.1 The exhibition

If a company is considering taking a stand at an exhibition, there are 5 key questions it should ask prior to making its decision:

1. How does attending the exhibition compliment the Marketing Objective?
2. Why is it felt necessary to go?
3. What does the company want to promote and/or sell?
4. Who is the target audience?
5. How much does it want to spend on the whole event?

These questions are laid out in section 10.1 of your workbook for you to complete, if this topic is currently applicable.

Some of the answers to these may include:

1. HOW:
1.1 The key promotional vehicle for the industry is its annual trade exhibition and therefore, to demonstrate firm market establishment, it is right to be present.
1.2 The company wishes to find out more about a particular industry and the market it services, therefore attending its major exhibition will provide

useful market research and/or expose the company to new customer groups.
1.3 Attendance at the exhibition is the flagship for the whole promotional campaign.

2. WHY
2.1 Provides the opportunity to liaise with a large number of existing and potential customers in one concentrated event.
2.2 Opportunity to announce the launch of a new product/service.
2.3 Looking to raise market awareness towards the presence of the company in the industry and generate new customer enquiries.

3. WHAT
3.1 Corporate identity
3.2 Product/service range.
3.3 Particular item.

4. AUDIENCE
4.1 Customer, consumer or both
4.2 Industrial, domestic or both
4.3 Level of media coverage the event is likely to attract.

5. BUDGET
Considerations include: Cost of the stand space; cost of manning the stand; cost of supporting promotional initiatives prior to, during and post the exhibition; cost of funding the support sales effort etc.

Section 10.2 of your workbook helps you to progress the initial thoughts you may have put down in section 10.1.

MARKET PROFILE

To support its objectives, the company will supplement its overall pricing policy with subtle techniques designed to help pull customers through the A.I.D.A.:

AWARENESS: Usage of loss leaders to attract the prospective customer's attention/awareness.
INTEREST: Stimulated through special offers, credit terms etc.
DESIRE: Encouraged through image pricing; ranging from a discount which makes for a good deal, through to ultra expensive to reinforce the exclusivity of the product etc.
ACTION: The final attractive special price that persuades the customer to make the deal/purchasing action immediately.

COMPETITORS (CURRENT AND POTENTIAL)

The table in 6.2 may also be used as a brand map.
A brand map enables a company to plot its pricing
position in relation to competitors, for example:

BRAND MAPPING

High

Premium strategy
xx
High value strategy

x

Rip off & false economy strategies

xx

x

Low quality   xx   Average strategies   x   High quality

Good value strategies
XX   XX

xx
x

Superb value strategies
xx

Economy strategies

Low price

The Xs denote competitors, which on your map
should also be named. The aim is to see where
there are fewer competitors and even gaps on the
map, looking at them making this your target for
development.

The "Safer" areas to focus on are those within the
tram lines, outside of the tram lines are short term
"Risk" approaches.

Use the Brand Map within section 6.2 of your
workbook to plot your competitor's positions.

DIFFERNTIALS

Whilst within its plan, a company may set down its
pricing objective and supporting policies for the
period under review, it must be prepared to
differentiate against these ideas, if there are
changes in the market; perhaps initiated by
unforeseen changes in competitors' activities,
increases in costs brought about by economic
change etc.

SETTING OUT OUR STRATEGY WITHIN A MARKETING PLAN

8.1 Why Plan?

In the average small business, where resources are
tight and the important issue is to spend time on
producing items and services for which there is a
buyer, there tends to be a natural reluctance to
spending time on planning and in particular,
formally documenting this planning.

However, if a business is compared to a machine,
then one expects that in order to get the best from
a machine, it is properly maintained and serviced
and, as it reaches the end of its useful life, is
scheduled for replacement. Progress this type of
attitude and one expects the machine to give good
reliable service and thereby yield a satisfactory
return on its investment.

Larger businesses usually follow the same approach. They develop a Business Plan which focuses on their development for the short, medium and long terms. Within their Business Plans, they incorporate a plan for Production, human Resources, Financial Management and Marketing; these topics may vary depending upon the nature of the business. By compiling such a plan, the larger business is establishing the direction in which it wants to go and the roads it will take to ensure its safe arrival.

All too often, the smaller business tends to take the attitude that planning is for the "Larger Boys" only and so takes a reactive approach to its development. This produces flaws in its management and approach and can lead to inefficiencies, frustration, late deliveries, loss of business and in the worst cases, closure of the company.

By taking time out to plan, the smaller business may also identify where it wants to get to and the route it will take to get there. This will help it to become more efficient, increase its chance of securing more work from existing customers and, develop new business. This will lead to various opportunities, such as developing additional businesses and/or take over from another organisation, thereby providing the owner(s) with a financial bonus and new opportunities.

The discipline of good planning provides another marketing tool, with reference to being able to demonstrate to existing customers that the businesses is capable of taking more work from them or illustrating to new customers, the capability of being able to handle large contracts.

Many owner/managers of small businesses would argue that they do plan but, that they do not formally document their plans. The problem with this is that should they suddenly be taken away from the business for an extended period of time, i.e. through a major illness etc., then those left to cope with the business in their absence, may lead the business in completely the wrong direction. Furthermore, the conveying of one's intentions to one's employees, through the production of a plan, helps them to understand the contribution they are expected to make in helping the business to fulfil its objectives and so, helps to give them greater job satisfaction, which in turn, usually has the effect of increasing their output at work.

Finally, the failure to formally document one's intentions puts further pressure on the mind to hold together the idea alongside current work pressures. The consequence is that all too often, crises push out the plans and so they fail to be put into action.

Owner/managers of smaller businesses are frequently reluctant to produce a plan because they feel obliged to produce a large, thick document, which they will never have time to refer to, thereby making the exercise pointless. A plan can be as large as one wants to make it and quite often, the most effective plan is the one which covers a single side of A4 and is posted on the office notice board for all to see, understand and aim to achieve.

The author would argue that owners/proprietors of smaller businesses should plan for the following reasons:

- ❖ To take time out of the daily routine to think through the following:
    - What does this business actually do?
    - Is it doing what was intended?
    - What should it be doing?
    - How should it be doing it?

Have a go at answering these in section 8 of your workbook.

- ❖ To communicate to themselves, their employees, successors and customers what it is that they intend doing with the business.
- ❖ To set a timetable for achieving their destination and so ensure that methods that need to be taken to ensure arrival are pursued within a given timescale.
- ❖ To establish a discipline for monitoring the progress of the business on a regular basis and so ensure that as the market changes, these changes are anticipated and, policies for reacting to them are installed in plenty of time.

Having focused so far on why a business should plan, attention is now turned towards what should be in the plan and how it may be presented.

8.2 Framework for a marketing plan:

As this publication is concerned with marketing, it only focuses on the elements of a Marketing Plan. There are other publications available which cover the topic of Business Planning in general.

There is no set formula for presentation, as every business is different and so may require variations on content etc. to suit its particular needs. However the author has found the following framework a trusty friend in helping her [is this a different author to the previous one who was a him?]to prepare plans for a variety of organisations across different industries and sizes.

Have you skipped that section?

Have you understood the text?

You might know more about business, but it's just like driving a car.

DO IT

Reality check

You need to make sure you are on the ground rather than in the air.

Do you know how much the cost of milk is or a loaf of bread? There are people who earn a great deal of money who do not. I worked with a chap call Vic Kithener: great man, but had no reality. Before I met him he was very high up in Wang, earning £20,000 per month (1990), he had people to do everything, clean, drive etc. his kitchen was spotless because he always ate out.

He was good with money but not reality. The same is in business: doing a business plan is easy. Doing one that stacks up is even easier (I have done plenty). However doing one that reflects both the business and reality is hard.

You have to be honest, if you are not - it's not the lender you are fooling, it's YOU. You see, if you budget for losses it's OK, but if you budget for increased profits that do not turn up then that's bad.

Look at companies for sale, they say put the owners' salary back in the business. You could but how many extra staff at what cost should you budget for? How key is the owner?

You have read about perception and reality. Well, it needs to be real for people to buy into it. Or it's just a concept that goes nowhere.

The truth about the internet

The internet was designed during the Cold War to be used as a communication tool. Much of this has been documented.

It has evolved into an information and disinformation tool. There are many scams on the net and as we are going to describe in viral marketing you can find out a great deal from the internet.

The internet is a doubled-edged sword, you need to offer the same product to all on the internet otherwise they will find out. Some retailers offer cheaper products on the net. This is because they have lower costs for this type of transaction.

The customer can in and out a great deal about your product ranges and therefore THEY decide when to buy. If you look at the PC market - promise your children a PC for Christmas but buy it in the New Year saving 10% - of if you know Intel are bringing out a new chip, buy it four weeks after this faster chip comes out because the older chips drop in price.

The internet can also change the way you interface in business. You can have a full report on the company or person within five minutes. You might still be talking to them on the phone.

You might be given a medical product, great; you can find out its side effects on the internet.

The only personal issue is that the internet is changing the way we communicate with each other. There is less done face to face and more in written form. This does not allow interaction.

Product demand can change like the wind, good and bad information can be found at the drop of a hat.

Viral marketing

Where to begin? Think of viral marketing as a virus!!!!

 It's a circle. Before 1500 AD, 99% of history was folk law, people around camp fires telling tales. was localised writing developed with people documenting facts and people, a sort of historic record.

Before the Industrial Revolution, the upper classes wrote letters, postcards etc. not that the middle class or working class could really read or write.

Post Industrial Revolution, papers could be produced and more people where reading.

After 2000, the internet became a tool.

You have 5 stages: let's look at them more closely in detail.

Media moved from one to one, to educated masses, to all masses, to one to one.

We sold our own vegetables, we sold our product to those who can read, we sold our product in supermarkets to the masses and we sold it on the net as an exclusive organic product.

The adoption of technology has increased. It took ten years for the train to go from the UK to America, seven years for VHS to take off, three years for DVD to reach the masses and eighteen months for MP3.

We adopt technology now without knowing it, your new mobile will have double the features of the last at a lesser price. Manufacturers and producers want you to consume, they add features to help this happen, however the reality is that their profits are in decline, not incline.

Viral marketing in effect takes us to where we started, in the global market we sell one to one. If you need facts on a product to purchase it, you look on the net.

Time to market is weeks and not years, you can produce in smaller volumes.

The product shift can take four hours rather than weeks or months. If a drug has bad press then people stop buying the same day.
MMR vaccination is a good example. It had bad press in 2005/ 2005 in the UK. The number of children having it fell. This in turn created an issue with the doctors, the impedance [unclear] is still waiting to happen.

You have 4 billion potential customers, who if they buy might buy direct or via your distribution channels. You have to have enough products to keep them happy but not enough to make the bank cry.

If people find a product cheaper in another country, they will buy it there. I saved 23% on a new car buying it on the internet,

Viral marketing helped *hotmail.com* come onto the market and get into the top five in a very short period of time. This cannot be under-estimated in its power.

You can do viral marketing, because you do. For every one person who is unhappy about a product, they tell twelve other people. It's a fact, what do you think of estate agents or banks?

I rest my case.

There will always be an England

The role of England has always been strange, while in Queen Victoria's day the sun did not set on the Empire, England still has a few ticks left.

When Margaret Thatcher was voted out of the party in 1984, there were many countries that wanted her and her reforms. Those reforms are challenging the very strong power houses of Europe, France and Germany. These countries are stuck in a mire of unemployment, bad working practices and heavy national debt.

Every nation will have its day, in biblical times it was Ethiopia, Egypt, Greece, then Rome (or Italy) then Genghis and his horde. The Industrial Revolution happened in the UK and the UK was an invader until after the Second World War, where Germany tried to take over (twice).

While the UK, is not liked throughout Europe, it still has a financial role to play in banking. The currency is fundamentally sound. However labour costs are high, employment is low. London is the most expensive capital for most things in Europe.

The recent bombing of London proved that there is a stiff upper lip; the people killed were not Caucasian (white) suited and booted people but rather normal people from a mixed race. England is not full of white faces, but rather is a mixed race culture.

My local Church of England school has 210 pupils where twenty-six do not have English as their first language. You might think this is a crap school? Well, the boys do better than the girls. Why? They want to be like their fathers, who are accountants, doctors and professionals: they have a dream.

This school is not on its own, however there are others where they are full of the same colour and have NO dreams, NO expectations and NO life.

You have got to have a dream, how otherwise can you have a dream come true?

They came from the East

In May 2004, there were 10 countries allowed into the EU. While NATO were happy, this changed the balance of power and landscape of the EU.

The old club of 12 were comfortable, however the large group had so many issues to address, it's no wonder why the French voted no.

The old club had the tiger economy of Ireland and the issues of Greece along with two power houses, France and Germany. The EU, created a currency that would help the common good. Which it did, and other countries wanted some of that action.

These countries will be the new tiger economies. They hold cheap and willing labour, with stable political policies while the average salary for Germany is €38,000, France €30,000 and Spain €18,000. These countries are up to 50% unemployed with more flexible labour with an average of €5,000.

They needed to join because they had always been part of a group. However they have similar issues to the old EU. The tiger economies are Lithuanian, Poland and Czech Republic. With issues in some of the other countries, [unclear] however these countries had fundamental issues to address. They have only been used to capitalism for 12 years and are still trying to cope with unemployment redundancy and alike. They are all proud people and even the unemployed clean the street.

A national paper owner at an embassy party put it like this, under Communism we had money but no goods and under Capitalism we have goods but no money. Many of these countries have had things they did not have for the last 50 years, they have reached their dreams.

They are however moving some factories from these countries to China as the wages are too high.

The 20 – 35 age group are highly educated and ready to work, however are often unable to work. All of these countries have been force to find flexible working conditions.

They are going to be the new power house of Europe.

Where is China?

At the time of writing China had still pegged its currency to the Dollar. Alan Greenspan had just delivered a talk in New York. There is pressure from the US to unpeg and devalue. The effect of this on the US economy is too much. The price of goods could rise by 20%, this giving inflation to the US economy. The producers would look to other Asian countries for cheap manufactured products.

China is known to be issuing 50% more RMB instruments that it should, but what Greenspan could not say was since these are pegged to the Dollar they are in effect building a Dollar reserve. This is worse for the US as 40% of all the bonds are helped by China and Japan. They need these countries to buy at least $78T in 2006.

China needs to be known; they have transformed their country, from subsistence to manufacturing. However the pain of growth is great, they are currently a net importer of raw material. They soon will be an exporter, steel as an example will move from 2007 from importer to exporter. Just watch the price fall.

On a human level, 30 years ago you would be asked when did you last eat? 10 years ago rice was the stable food, meat like chicken only for holidays. However now you have 1.4 billion people, all looking to eat every day. The average wage is a Dollar a day and two bowls of rice. However the consumer economy is so large everyone wants some of it.

Currently, there is not enough electricity for the country. The six regions are taking it in turns to go without it. This increase the amount of fuel purchased and has a knock-on effect on the economy.

Shanghai province, will soon challenge that of California. This will prove difficult for some governments to come to terms with.

What hope the world?

It's your world, you made the mess, please can you tidy it up?

There is war, famine, pollution and corruption. These things are all over the world. There are the natural resources that are being used up like there is no tomorrow. Greed and fear (already covered) are used to control the masses.

At the tender age of sixteen, I saw parts of the Far East before they started ripping it apart. You have been given this mess. Will you give a bigger issue to your next generation?

40% of homes in the UK are occupied by single people and while life expectancy increases, the need to consume everything, including each other, is worse than it ever was.

There is starting to be a shift of power, China might have the power that Japan dreamt of? Or will the USA still keep control of 1.4 billon people?

Not controlling carbon emissions might increase profit and kill customers; not treating water might sound fun but kill your workers. Look at the Rhine. It starts crystal clear in the Swiss Alps and after passing three countries it flows into the sea. Almost every mile they take some water out and put it back in a worst state. The people need this water to drink, for farming, for industry. But they are without doubt polluting it.

You have the power of one (covered earlier) therefore your vote counts. The difference that you can make is so vast. It might be adopting a child or the giving of aid but in 100 years, unless we are in space, this point is going to be unliveable for another 400 million years.

Europe, the bigger picture

Europe for many has moved from the common market to this group of 25 countries that all need each other to fight against (in trade terms) other groups.

Countries outside the current Euro zone want to get in, while countries that are in want to get out. There is too much in fighting and the need to solve the common issues often left behind.

You can operate in most of the countries but you will find that some countries will be cheaper and tax free. You must consider that there is no common language among the countries. They are like the USA with no common tax. Iin mainland Europe people and businesses do migrate to suit their needs.

Comply with the basic requirement, you might have to have 25 serviced offices (they hate ringing outside their own country), you will need staff that can really talk the same LOCAL language and you need to solve those very nasty distribution problems. While the banking system is great, the fundamentals need addressing.

The powerhouses of Europe are down at the moment (Germany & France) due to strict labour laws. Once they are up and running, the European economy should be better off. However with unemployment at 10% compared to under 5% in the UK and Ireland. They will have some time before they can regain control.

The countries are not polarised into one extra, they are both extremes. They have though a common need.

I do not think that Europe can last in its current state, the No vote will see to that. The need is for reform but how this is now done is for others.

The same is true of Europe as with the USA, find a friendly state and start there. The currency should be stable.

USA and the inside track

The USA is a great market, however governed by 50 plus different laws. Only 20% of the population have passports. You must budget to get into this market then double the amount you expect to spend.

The amount of litigation is vast; you must have good cover on your service or product. If you are not covered you could lose it all.

This is a do-or-die country. Do it and you will have an income, don't and you could die. Fashion can change in days; it is different from state to state.

To enter the US market or to stay in it you need to constantly reinvent yourself.

If you do not have deep pockets or the desire to tame the US market then just sell your product on the internet to this market.

They are great people and a few percentage points of the total market will make you big bucks. However the cost of going into this market might be too big.

There are many products to sell, but you are better involving your customers in this market or even buying an existing business rather than going into it.

They are the easiest market to approach. You have over 360 million people understanding a common tongue. You, as always, need to start in one state. Choose the easiest for your product, then role [roll?] out.

The international policies are great as are the needs of the people. The move is to better fuel efficient cars and modes of transports. There is also a great divider of rich and poor.

They consume almost everything, while having great natural resources themselves they buy in a high volume of overseas product.s

Marketing

If we knew what worked we would not waste the rest of our money on.[word missing?]

There are different ways, you must understand your customer, whether B2C or B2B. What are their buying patterns, what do they like to buy?

As discussed in viral marketing we are moving to an individual purchase. Tesco have poured millions into their club card, they have the software to identify what their individual buys. This is the type of data we are taking about.

Everything comes in cycles, just like the seasons of the year. Fashions keep on coming back, and there is always a different form of new media.

The issue of marketing is whether it's better to do none than do the wrong form of marketing.

You could hire an expensive team that are crap, or do it yourself more effectively. The tool section of the book should help you. If you get a consultant in, then ask for two hours free, then a written brief. Take this brief and do as much of it as you can.

The best long term marketing campaign was also the worst.

New Coke was for the new generation, it cost the company $100m, but the profile raised the brand.

Sure it was shit and no one liked it, but the customer (to whom you market) demanded old Coke back. They had interaction with the customer, this is what you need in marketing.

You can't market safe sex to the over 80s, or bed pants to the under 25s. Be careful of your marketing, careful that you are targeting the correct people. You might find that referrals work far better than marketing.

It is better to send out nothing than send out crap. The person getting your marketing material will have a dim view of you.

Be careful, do not be the first or the last to market. If you are the first to try a new marketing campaign, they will use you to learn how to do it, if you are the last then the market will be saturated.

You could be marketing yourself, but are you marketable?

Meeting about meetings

Be a man of action. What is the purpose of the meeting?

We have already discussed consultants and meetings, try and stay out of these. If you go, opt in for the jobs for which you will be effective. Where the meeting is high level and you know the grass roots stuff, then all you need to do is fill in the holes: you can do this effectively.

I once did some constancy, [consultancy?]for a £35m manufacturer of good standing. They would ring up every other week saying that they had urgent news. Once I had travelled 150 miles; I found out it was only to have a chat.

I arranged a sales call (but called it a satisfaction meeting) with a big broker, every week on this day not only did I leave with many orders but also knew his production schedule.

Unproductive meetings waste time, and time is not something you can have back. Ask to see the agenda for the meeting. If there is not an agenda submit your own, if they do not accept it then you might refuse to go.

Control the meeting, directly or indirectly, if you do not agree then "pass", if you do not understand - ask them to explain.

By not being invited to meetings you are not in the loop, where you are in the meeting take your own notes as the minutes might not be a true reflection on the meeting.

I worked in a company where the CEO took delight in adjusting the minutes of a sales meeting to reflect his greatness.

Where you have no faith in the chair of the meeting or the direction you or the other attendees will talk over the chairman's direction or even just not turn up.

At one company I worked for we had bacon sandwiches at the meeting: this soon lost its appeal after seven meetings. Do not go unless you can add value or you need to know something about the subject.

By being informed and directive you need not take up the chair role to steer the meeting but rather keep things going because of what you know.

Do one well or 90 badly?

Would you prefer to do one job well? Or 90 badly?

This is the issue in today's environment, it's easy to do 90 jobs but to do one well is better. You can't afford to be jack of all trades and master of none.

You can learn new skills but you will find that once you have one skill the others will be easy to do.

As you learn ONE skill you will be a true master, as you progress to learning something different many of the skills will be similar. A child only learns to walk once or write once. When moving to a country with a different tongue the letters are the same, it's only the meaning that has changed. [not true. Hebrew, Arabic etc.]

If you can't read or write in your native tongue what hope have you got with this new language?

When going to an interview they might ask for strengths and weaknesses. You are better off having good employable strengths than a heap of weaknesses.

Play to your strengths and get others to cover your weaknesses, you will find if you are a hyper maniac then you WILL be strong.

Hyper mania what now?

Welcome to the point that starts making sense.

Your life is just that: your life.

You need to take control of it; there are plenty of people out there to help.

Have your trusted contacts and that's it, no more, just them.

Read the other books and live life to the full.

Profile worker

Your life as a hyper manic will be a constant move from job to job, thing to thing.

You will find however that you start to build up a bank of contacts where you have not burnt the bridges. Often these people will want to keep in touch with you to find out what is going on.

While for the hypo manic, life is full of extremes. You will be chasing old contacts that you have dumped on, while even the bank could be chasing you.

THINK TWICE THEN ACT!

Reality check

Your need to do this yourself; find someone you can trust to talk about it.

Sorry if you are a hypo maniac, just go for it. The answers were in the book. Have fun.

That action plan

Your need is to plan, don't just leave work.

Plan, think about what you do and what you like, then go and do it.

Mania is great - such a high without drugs.

Revisit your action plan every week and think about what you need to learn.

Save money, but above everything, enjoy LIFE.

Coming to terms with hyper mania

Your life might make more sense now.

The fact of you leaving all that disaster behind you or the wondering what life is about.

Come to terms with it, don't fear it. Embrace it, for your purpose it has been revealed.

These so real dreams that you can't forget, do not let them worry you but look forward to them.

Sure you might get low, but you are probably the best salesman of the company.

Now you begin to understand, go, get them tiger.

I need help!!

Your life might start to make sense now, not that they will come and lock you up.

But rather, you will start to control more of your everyday experience, what you do and how you do it.

Once you decide to change, the rest is easy.

Help? No - understanding and love.

Read Hyper Mania Explained with full detail from experts on the subject covered

You are either coming to terms with what you have or with what someone else has.

Yes, this is rather hard; there are two further books on the subject.

Hyper mania Explained gives an in-depth analysis of the text in this book. It's ideal for those who seek more information for themselves and for their loved ones.

Published by chipmunkapublishing

Do you get it yet? Gives a blow by blow of mania. This pulls no punches and expect no prisoners. This book has been written by an ex-hyper maniac and a bipolar. These people set up Chipmunka to help save the world. It might just open your eyes or the eyes of your loved one.

Published by Chipmunkapublishing

Postscript

Understand your life or be a bystander: the choice is yours……..

YOU are loved
You are special
You are you
You need direction
You need faith
You can do it
You are the only thing holding you back every day

You have POWER, Love and self control: Hyper maniac

You have power: Hypomaniac

Hypo maniac learn,
Be stronger
Understand
And then have love
For as Rome was not built in a day you need patience.

www.ingramcontent.com/pod-product-compliance
Lightning Source LLC
Chambersburg PA
CBHW031200270326
41931CB00006B/349